Nutrition For Healthy Kids

You Are What You Eat
Part 1

2nd EDITION

JENNIFER NEEDHAM, MS

Copyright © 2014 Jennifer Needham

All rights reserved.

ISBN-13: 978-1501031014
ISBN-10: 1501031015

For MARAALCASSLJ. You are my world.

CONTENTS

Lesson 1 - Organic Taste Test   1

Lesson 2 - PLU Codes   5

Lesson 3 - Genetically Modified Foods   9

Lesson 4 - USDA Organic   13

Lesson 5 - Sweeteners – Splenda   17

Lesson 6 - Sweeteners – Aspartame   22

Lesson 7 - Sweeteners - High Fructose Corn Syrup   26

Lesson 8 - Produce - From Seed to Table   31

Lesson 9 - Produce - Basic Botany of Edible Plants   35

Lesson 10 - Sustainable Farming   39

Lesson 11 - Meat - Grass fed and Pastured Meats   43

Lesson 12 - Meat - Life Cycles and Animal Husbandry Basics   47

Lesson 13 - Dairy - What is Pasteurization?   51

Lesson 14 - Dairy - Cheese, Butter, Milk, Curds & Whey, Buttermilk, and Yogurt   55

Lesson 15 – Eggs   58

Answers to lessons 1-15   62

Introduction and Statement of Purpose

There is a lack of curricula available for elementary students to learn about nutrition from an integrated nutrition perspective. Millions of dollars have been spent by governments, corporations, and schools nationwide to develop appropriate materials to teach children about nutrition. However, by and large these programs teach nutrition from a traditional perspective of nutrients, digestion, counting calories, and learning about the food groups. One ubiquitous example of this is the Choose My Plate initiative put forth by the U.S. Department of Agriculture. These programs teach the chosen material well, but don't go far enough to create critical thinking skills in kids who need to learn more than what's being presented to truly be healthy.

Literature Review and Rationale for Research

There is no published, peer-reviewed research on the topic of teaching integrative nutrition principles to children. A search for an organized and structured curriculum to review for this purpose was also not successful.

Many cities have community gardens where residents work cooperatively to grow their own food, and occasionally volunteers are utilized to offer training sessions and basic "how to plant a seed" classes for kids. Some historical sites or municipal recreation departments offer seasonal opportunities for children to learn how to milk a cow, or how farmers harvest corn, for example. But these types of programs only speak about sustainability, ecology, and perhaps saving money on grocery budgets; there is no talk of nutrition or why it is healthier to live without chemicals or avoiding food produced on a mass scale.

A curriculum for children is needed that teaches more peripheral aspects of nutrition that are often not covered by mainstream education. How food is produced greatly impacts its nutritional value. This project will use an information-based approach that provides the other side of the story that kids and their families are not learning from school health classes and public health resources.

Project Objectives

The objectives of the Nutrition for Healthy Kids curriculum are:

1. Promotion of critical thinking skills in making nutrition choices – It is one thing to learn that vegetables are good for you and trans-fats are not, and quite another to understand *why*.

2. Application of knowledge learned to real life – Live it! Kids need to be able to apply their nutrition knowledge to other foods and new situations.

3. To target the nutrition lessons to a homeschooling audience – The program is not targeted to specific grades or ages, but to general ranges of kids and their abilities. Homeschooling families often have multiple children and this curriculum seeks to offer something to each of them. It will be easily adjusted to different ages by allowing parents to increase or decrease the level of complexity of each topic addressed. Above all, it will provide a service to homeschooling families, both through the education of their children and also sharing the lessons learned with the rest of the family.

4. Appealing to all types of learners – Most visual learners excel at traditional schoolwork, while auditory and kinesthetic learners suffer. This curriculum seeks to provide "something for everyone", so all children can benefit from the lessons, regardless of their learning style.

5. Efficiency – brief lessons with a minimum of prep time – The lessons can be accomplished in 20-30 minutes a week, with little required prep time and few materials to buy. Answers are provided for all worksheets to cut down on time spent grading assignments.

6. Providing optional worksheets for those who want to use them – For those homeschooling families who are interested in reinforcing the lessons with written assignments, or to have a written record of the work for a homeschool portfolio, these worksheets and answer keys are provided with each lesson.

FOR FAMILIES: USE OF THE PROGRAM

This is intended as a resource for homeschooling families who seek to include nutrition lessons in their curriculum. Because it is intended to serve a wide audience of homeschoolers, this course can be easily adjusted to different ages by allowing parents to increase or decrease the granularity of the material. Parents should preview the lessons to determine the best way to present the material to their families.

Please do not mass-distribute the lessons, worksheets, or other information presented, although you are welcome to copy the materials for use within your own household. If you wish to use these materials in a co-op or classroom setting, please contact the owner, through NutritionForHealthyKids.com, to obtain permission. Nutrition For Healthy Kids content may not be used in any for-profit manner.

DISCLAIMER

While all of the information presented is believed to be accurate, it is not absolutely guaranteed. Please do your own research on the topics discussed and make your own decisions. Feedback and suggested corrections are welcome if you find some bit of information to be in error. Nothing here is intended as medical advice or to replace the treatment or recommendations of your doctor or other health professional.

By using NutritionForHealthyKids.com and/or accompanying assignments, texts, and worksheets, you consent to hold the site, Nutrition for Healthy Kids, its owner, and all subsidiaries and representatives harmless from any and all repercussions, damages, or liability.

LESSON 1: ORGANIC TASTE TEST

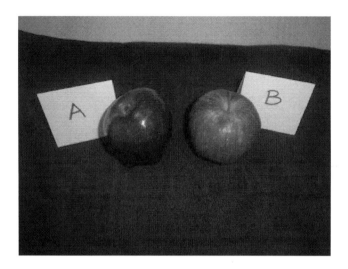

This is a great, short activity to be done at snack time, and it's wonderful for involving the whole family. Kids of all ages enjoy it!

You probably know that organic produce costs more than its conventionally grown counterparts, but many people feel that higher price is justified [1]. Some studies do show that organic foods are better for us and offer health benefits above conventionally grown foods [2]. Are you willing to pay more for organic foods?

What's the difference between organic and non-organic?

(Note to parents: Before you start, ask your kids to write down what they think organic means. This is a helpful pretest to refer to after the lesson so you see what they learned. The answers they give you will, of course, depend on where on the nutrition spectrum your family is, and whether or not your kids have been exposed to organic foods. But don't worry, there are no wrong answers! When that's done, you can discuss with your children some of the explanations below, so they have some knowledge about organic produce.)

What makes something "organic"?

    A) Organic produce is not sprayed with chemical pesticides and is not fertilized with chemical fertilizers [3]. This is important because those chemicals are difficult to wash off, and people will inadvertently ingest some of them when they eat the produce. Some of these chemicals are actually formulated to resist being washed off the plants by rain, which makes them difficult to wash off in your kitchen sink too! Yuck - who wants to *eat* stuff designed to kill bugs?

B) Organic produce is largely farmed using sustainable methods that are healthier for the crops and the environment in general. There are strict rules about what types of natural fertilizers can be used, and companion planting, barriers to pests, and old-fashioned weed-pulling are utilized to avoid the need for chemicals [3].

C) One big difference with organic foods is that they are never genetically modified [3]. What's that? It's when scientists insert foreign DNA (sometimes even from an animal!) into a plant's DNA in order to confer certain favorable characteristics to that plant's offspring. Not all of the long-term effects of human consumption of GMOs (genetically modified organisms) are known, simply because they haven't been around long enough yet [4].

But mice and other lab animals have much shorter life spans than humans, so the effects of a GMO diet across the lifespan have been documented in these animals. The results are striking. There's an increased rate of infertility in animals fed a GMO diet [5], and allergies to various foods and other compounds seem to be much higher in these animals as well [6,7]. In general, animals consuming GMOs have shorter life spans and more health problems [8].

D) It has also been demonstrated that in many cases organic foods contain higher levels of nutrients than their conventionally-grown counterparts. An organic fruit, for example, may contain more of certain vitamins than a non-organic fruit of the same type and size [9] and organic milk contains more omega-3 fatty acids than the non organic version [10].

Let's start the taste test!

1. You'll need two apples of the same variety, one organic and one not. I used red delicious apples because they're readily available. Label one "A" and one "B".

2. Let the kids pass them around to inspect them, and make a list of their observations. Which one has a deeper color? Which is heavier? Shinier? More uniformly shaped? Even young children can come up with some great observations!

3. Have the kids think it over, and based on what they've learned about organics, decide which apple they think is the organic one. Write down the results and the justifications on the worksheet included with this lesson.

4. Next, slice the apples and have everyone try a bite of each. Again, write down any observations. Besides the subjective question of which tastes better, try to decide objectively which is juicier, and how the color inside differs, how many seeds are present, etc. Do some detective work!

5. Ask the kids if tasting the apples changed their opinion of which one is organic.

6. And the organic apple is....drumroll please....Reveal the organic apple and see who was right!

To stretch the lesson, you could also have your child create graphs or tables of the data they collected, or turn it into a full science experiment by following the scientific method to create and test a hypothesis about which apple is organic. An essay idea for older kids would be "Pros and Cons of Eating Organic Foods", and they could also do more research on GMOs or sustainable farming methods, for example. Have some fun with it!

Finally, are you wondering which apple is organic in the above picture?
"B" is the organic one.
Happy taste-testing!

As you work through this activity, answer the questions on the next page.

PRE-TEST QUESTION:
What does "organic" mean? Something else to think about is whether or not you think you'd like the organic apple better *if you knew in advance it was organic.* Of course, this would defeat the purpose of having a taste test, but it's true that sometimes people have made up their minds about a food before they've even tried it. Do you think you'd like an organic apple, or does it sound new and scary to you? Some groups in the food industry pay lots of money for surveys and consumer studies to predict which flavors, textures, and descriptions of food people will likely buy [11].

POST-TEST ASSIGNMENT:
True or False

1. T / F Sustainable farming is healthier for the environment than conventional farming.

2. T / F Chemical pesticides sprayed on crops are easily washed off in your kitchen.

3. T / F In many cases, organic foods contain higher levels of nutrients than their conventionally-grown counterparts.

4. T / F In scientific experiments, lab animals fed a diet of GMO foods grew up healthier and lived longer than similar animals who did not eat GMO foods.

5. T / F When growing organic berries, putting netting around the berries to keep birds from eating them is an acceptable way to protect the berry harvest.

ACTIVITY:
What variety of apples are you using?

What are your observations about the apples?

Based upon these observations, which one do you think is organic?   Why?

After tasting the apples, which one do you think tastes better? Does this change your mind about which one is organic?

Write down any additional observations you've made about the apples after cutting and tasting them.

What is your final answer? Which is the organic apple? Compile your observations in this data table to help you decide.

	Apple A	Apple B
color		
shape		
size		
smell		
taste		
seeds		
other		
other		

Did you choose the organic apple correctly? _____

ADDITIONAL EXERCISES:

During your next shopping trip, compare the price of organic apples and non-organic apples. Which costs more? Why do you think it costs more?

LESSON 2: PLU CODES

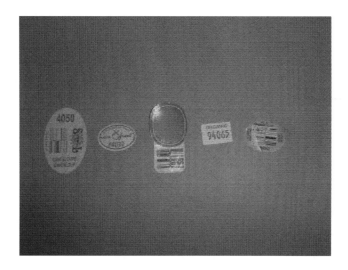

This lesson explores those tiny numbered stickers you find on produce at the grocery store. **They're called PLU codes, which stands for "price-look-up"**, and there are over 1400 different codes [1]. Talk to your kids about how the cashier at the store weighs the produce and enters the PLU code at the cash register. This is how the computerized cash register knows how much to charge you for that item.

In addition, **PLU codes help stores keep track of inventory**. When you buy 2 pounds of bananas, the store knows its supply of "4011 bananas" just decreased by 2 pounds. The ease of check-out and the inventory features are the reasons PLU codes were created. They make life a little easier for retailers selling produce, and this is the incentive suppliers have to keep using PLU codes. This system is very beneficial to retailers, so they prefer to buy their produce from suppliers who have already gone to the trouble of classifying their items and labeling them with PLU codes.

PLU codes were never intended for consumers to use. They were created by the International Federation for Produce Standard (IFPS), and meant to ease the relationship between suppliers and retailers [1]. However, saavy consumers can gain some valuable information about the produce they buy by using PLU codes themselves.

PLU codes are usually 4 digit numbers beginning with either a 3 or 4. To code the product as organic, a number 9 is added to the beginning. To code the product as genetically-modified (GMO), an 8 is added to the beginning. These are clues consumers can look for when shopping.

But it isn't foolproof. Remember that it is advantageous to suppliers and retailers to label organic products differently, with a number 9 [1]. If they are labeled differently, it is easier to charge more for them, so **there is an incentive for organic products to be labeled with a 9.**

However, countless studies and surveys have shown that people prefer NOT to eat genetically-modified foods if they can help it [2]. Suppliers and retailers know that foods labeled as GMO will likely not sell as well as their conventional or organic counterparts, so the concept of **labeling GMO foods is actually a DISINCENTIVE to sales**.

Since using **the PLU system is not mandatory or regulated by law in most areas**, many suppliers of GMO produce choose not to label their items as GMO. They'll get better sales if people can't tell they're buying GMO. **Therefore, while organic products are usually labeled with a 9, genetically modified products *are not always labeled* with an 8**. This is a great opportunity to introduce the concept of marketing to your kids! How can you best sell the product? By telling people what is really in it....or not?

Another important point to make is that PLU codes are only used for produce that needs to be weighed. Usually this means fruits and vegetables sold by the pound. Prepackaged produce, like berries in plastic containers, or a 5 pound bag of potatoes, will have a UPC code (a barcode) for scanning, rather than a PLU code. It's all about making things easier for the retailer. If they can find a way to put a UPC code on something, that's certainly easier for them than having to weigh the produce and enter a PLU code, right?

ACTIVITY:

This lesson would lend itself well to a trip to the store to check out the produce section. See if you can find some organic produce, beginning with a 9. It will be much more difficult to find GMO products, beginning with an 8! Write down the products and codes you found:

Examine the table of PLU codes on the next page, which is a modified selection copied from a spreadsheet of PLU codes from the Produce Marketing Association.(Source:http://www.plucodes.com/Default.aspx) [3]. Keeping in mind what we've learned about PLU codes, answer the following questions.

1. What is the code for pumpkin?

2. What is the code for organic bananas?

3. Which type of apple has the code 4182?

4. What color of rhubarb is listed?

5. What is the code for limes?

6. Why does the code for plumcot begin with an 8?

7. List two organic products found on the spreadsheet.

8. What is the code for genetically modified corn?

9. What is the code for organic white peaches?

10. What is the code for large, tree-ripened asparagus?

PLU CODES [3]

Code	Item		
4179	APPLES	Satsuma	Citrus unshiu
4182	APPLES	Sharlin	Cucumis melo
4522	ASPARAGUS	Tree Ripened	Small Prunus ssp
4523	ASPARAGUS	Tree Ripened	Large Prunus ssp
4011	BANANAS	Wood Ear	Auricularia auricula
94011	BANANAS	Wood Ear	Auricularia auricula
3273	BEETS	Crimson/Majestic	Vitis vinifera
83087	CORN	General Leclerc	Pyrus spp.
3337	FIGS	Zucchini/Courgette	C.pepo Round
3098	LETTUCE	Medium	Punica granatum
4048	LIMES	Red Solanum	tuberosum
94400	PEACHES	White	C.pepo
4673	PEAS	Helianthus annus	
83611	PLUMCOT	interspecific plum	Arachis hypogaea
3133	PUMPKIN	White - mini	Cucurbita pepo
4658	ONIONS	Borago officinalis	
4742	RADISH	Oyster Pleuotus	ostreatus
4745	RHUBARB	Red	Ribes sativum
4091	SWEETPOTATO	White	Ipomoea batato
4812	TURNIP	White	Allium spp.
4945	WALNUTS	Treviso	Cichorium intybus

CRITICAL THINKING QUESTIONS:

1. A woman bought 2 pounds of white, seedless grapes on sale for 99 cents per pound. Would you expect the grapes to have a PLU code or UPC code?

2. Imagine you found corn you wanted to buy at the grocery store, and it had a four-digit PLU code. What does this mean? Is it conventional? Organic? GMO? Can you determine this for sure?

LESSON 3: GENETICALLY-MODIFIED FOODS

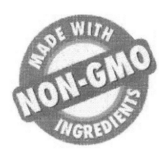

The topic of genetically modified foods (or GMO, genetically modified organisms) is one of the scariest things our society is faced with. GMOs are EXTREMELY unhealthy!

What are the problems with GMO foods?

GMO foods were once touted as revolutionary science, the wondrous result of years of study and research in genetic engineering. GMOs were going to give us super-foods, packed full of better nutrient content, and make healthier foods more widely available. What has actually happened, however, is that genetic engineering has been used to produce foods resistant to many known plant diseases and pests. One way of looking at it is that genetic engineering allows growers to get their product to the marketplace quicker and more cheaply, which makes their business more profitable. The process involves scientists inserting foreign DNA (often animal or bacterial) into a plant's DNA in order to confer certain favorable characteristics to that plant's offspring[1].

Some GMO seed companies have restricted access to their seeds for scientists who wish to study them, preferring to only allow studies that reflect favorably on GMOs to be conducted[2,3]. Because of this, it's hard to know what sources of information to trust regarding the safety of genetically modified foods. It's important to realize that the FDA approved GMO foods for human consumption without requiring safety testing on humans to be performed, and instead classifying GMOs as "generally recognized as safe" because their nutrient content is *assumed* to be similar to comparable non-GMO foods[4]. Numerous studies performed on lab animals fed a GMO diet, however, resulted in some striking findings. Lab animals who consume GMOs have a higher percentage of[5]

1. allergies, sensitivity to other foods, immune reactions
2. liver atrophy, toxicity, dysfunction
3. infertility and reproductive abnormalities, lower birth weights, higher infant mortality
4. general rates of disease and poor health

Why do GMO crops have these effects?

It is suspected that much of the damage from eating GMOs results from other genetic changes that occur when the foreign DNA is spliced into the plant's DNA. This process is not a smooth fit, and *results in hundreds to thousands of unpredictable mutations* in completely unrelated sections of the plant's DNA[6].

Remember, this is a very different process from natural breeding, and when these GMO plants reproduce, they are passing along these mutations from damaged DNA right along with the more "favorable" ability to resist pesticide, or whatever other traits have been spliced into their genetic information[6]. Think of it as collateral damage resulting from the genetic engineering process.

The human body has never before had to deal with foreign DNA injected into its food supply, much less foreign DNA that contains literally thousands of potentially dangerous mutations. No wonder there are side effects!

What crops are genetically modified?

This is subject to change, but there are currently 5 major genetically-modified crops being grown for food in the United States.
1. soy
2. corn
3. canola
4. cotton (This can be a food crop because it is used to produce cottonseed oil.)
5. sugar beets

In addition, smaller percentages of other crops are also GMO, such as yellow crookneck squash, papaya, and zucchini. There is a long list of GMO crops included in the "answers" section for this lesson.

What qualities are transferred to plants by genetically modifying them?

There are any number of qualities that farmers would find useful in their crops. Some plants are made resistant to specific plant diseases known to affect them, or to produce fruit years earlier than normal, and others are made more drought-tolerant or able to survive despite massive doses of weed-killer[7]. There is a variety of GMO corn known as Bt-corn because it is deliberately infected with a bacteria that causes its cells to produce their own Bt pesticide[8]. The corn plant actually produces its own pesticide!

How can I tell if food is genetically modified?

The easiest way to avoid GMO is to either grow the food yourself, buy from a local farmer you trust, or buy foods labeled as USDA organic. Organic foods never contain GMOs.

Otherwise, if a food doesn't specifically say on the package "non-GMO", there is no way to know for sure. In most areas, producers are not required to label their GMO foods, and most choose not to do so.

But if you want to avoid GMOs, here are some tips. More than 90% of the corn and soy grown in the United States is GMO. If a food contains corn or soy, odds are it is GMO. This includes a multitude of foods containing high fructose corn syrup!

Also, the growth hormone often given to dairy cows, rBST, is genetically modified, and makes its way into the milk these animals produce[9]. The FDA has come out with an official position that rBST milk does not differ from non-rBST milk, but many scientists find fault with this statement[10]. At any rate, if you want to avoid GMOs, you need to avoid rBST. Organic dairy never contains rBST, and there are certain brands of non-organic dairy that do not use it, but this will require some research on your part.

GMOs are everywhere. They are rapidly contaminating more and more of our food supply, and they're increasingly difficult to avoid. One survey of teenagers found that while their knowledge of the facts about GMOs was weak, they tended to distrust the motives of food companies trying to market GMO foods as safe[11]. What do *you* think?

ACTIVITY:

Take a trip into your kitchen to play detective! Look in the refrigerator and pantry to see how many GMO products you can find. Even if your family tries to eat organically, you may be surprised at how many GMOs sneak into your diet! Write down what items you find, and why you think they're GMO.

The group GMOInside.org has some fun, free labels you can use. (or you can make your own labels!) You can find instructions on how to download and print their labels here http://gmoinside.org/launch-labels/

It might be fun to bring some of these labels into the kitchen to search for GMO ingredients in your pantry. Put a label on the GMO foods you discover!

Here's something worthy of a family discussion: Do you think there should be mandatory labeling of GMO products in the stores? Do customers have a right to know if the products they buy are GMO? Why or why not?

True or False

1. T / F The growth hormone rBST given to dairy cows is GMO.

2. T / F One of the effects of a GMO diet seen in lab animals is infertility.

3. T / F Yellow crookneck squash, papaya, and zucchini are safe to eat because the FDA will not allow them to be genetically modified.

4. T / F High fructose corn syrup is most often made from non-GMO corn.

5. T / F Genetically modified produce is always labeled with a PLU code that begins with 8.

Short answer questions

1. Name at least three food crops in the U.S. that are commonly genetically modified.

2. Name at least one physical effect observed in lab animals fed a GMO diet.

Additional research topics for advanced students:

1. The FDA approved the use of GMOs in our food supply in 1992, when the FDA official spearheading this policy was Michael Taylor, former vice president of biotech & agriculture company Monsanto. Do some research online about Monsanto and write about whether or not you think putting Michael Taylor in charge of this effort at the FDA created a conflict of interest.

2. What are terminator seeds?

3. Do some research on your own and read more about genetically engineered animals. Discuss your findings with your family. Here is one suggestion to get you started:

Fish, pigs, and mosquitoes: Genetic engineering in animals (http://www.gmo-safety.eu/basic-info/1301.transgene-tiere.html)

Critical thinking and discussion for advanced students:

According to a 2004 study published in *Nature Biotechnology*[12], some bacteria from GMO soy have shown the ability to transfer into human intestinal cells and continue functioning there.

Some types of GMO corn have the ability to produce their own pesticide, to keep insects at bay. If something like this were to take up residence in the human intestinal tract, what would be the result?

LESSON 4: USDA ORGANIC

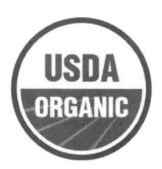

How do you know if something is organic? The National Organic Program, which is implemented by the USDA, specifies exactly what it takes to be organic[1].

- no synthetic fertilizers
- no GMO (genetically modified organisms) in seeds
- no synthetic pesticides
- no synthetic growth hormones in livestock
- no antibiotics given to livestock
- no food irradiation

It's important to note, however, that organic farming of produce and livestock has grown into a big business. Much of the organic product in grocery stores still comes from large farms, just ones that follow organic practices.

If you want to buy from small farmers, your best bet is to buy from local sources, such as your area's farmers' market. Then you can just *ask* the farmer what they spray on their crops, or if their seed is genetically modified, etc. There is a lot of additional paperwork involved in certifying your crops as organic, and fees to pay for the approval process as well, so many smaller farms cannot afford to become certified even though they may follow organic practices. It's worth asking at the farmers' market if they follow organic practices but aren't certified. If you trust the farmer you buy from, you could get organic, local food for less money.

For larger organic producers, oversight from the USDA's National Organic Program ensures they follow organic methods. If something is certified organic, it will have the "USDA Organic" emblem on it. The certification process was intended to protect consumers by standardizing the term organic. **If a product does not have the USDA Organic seal, it has not been through the certification process.** Some food packages may say things like "made with organic corn", and while this claim *may* be true, unless a product has the USDA Organic seal, there has been no oversight to verify the organic claims[2]. Buyer beware!

A product whose ingredients are 95% or more organic can be labeled "organic" and carry the USDA Organic seal. If a product contains between 70-94% organic ingredients, it can be labeled "contains organic ingredients"[2].

There is an important distinction to be made between the USDA providing oversight to the certification process and the independent third parties who agree to follow the USDA guidelines and certify products as organic.

Who Certifies That Organic Foods Follow USDA Guidelines?
The first picture below is a can of organic cooking spray and a jar of organic blackberry-applesauce. They both have the USDA Organic seal on their packaging. The second picture is the back of the can, where you can see the words "Certified Organic By QAI". That's the organization empowered by the USDA to certify products who follow the USDA's guidelines for organic. The last picture is the back of the applesauce jar, which says "Certified Organic by the Washington State Department of Agriculture". These are just two examples, but there are many other organizations who actually do the certifying on behalf of the USDA[3].

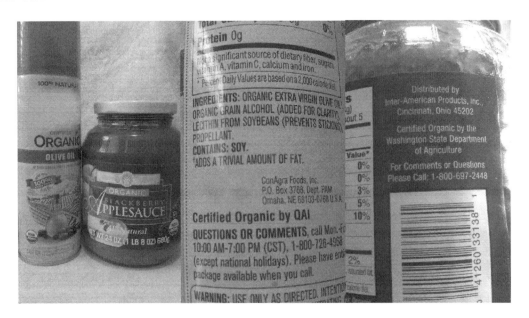

Watch this short video about the USDA National Organic Program. It is called "What Does The USDA Organic Label Really Mean?" You can search YouTube for it or try this link:
http://youtu.be/CIgt9JtCeQ8

(If you want to read more about the National Organic Program, you can visit their website at http://www.ams.usda.gov/AMSv1.0/nop.)

True or False

1. T / F The National Organic Program is administered by the FDA, which regulates what foods carry the USDA Organic seal.

2. T / F The National Organic Program regulates the standards for any farm, wild crop harvesting, or handling operation that wants to sell an agricultural product as organically produced.

3. T / F If a package of taco shells contains organic corn but GMO canola oil, it can be certified organic.

4. T / F Organic standards do not allow chemicals to be used on produce when it is grown, but after the plants are harvested, they can be irradiated to kill microorganisms.

5. T / F Livestock raised according to organic standards cannot be given antibiotics or growth hormones.

DISCUSSION:
Look back through what you've learned. Why are organic foods healthier?

Label-Reading: Which products below are USDA Organic?

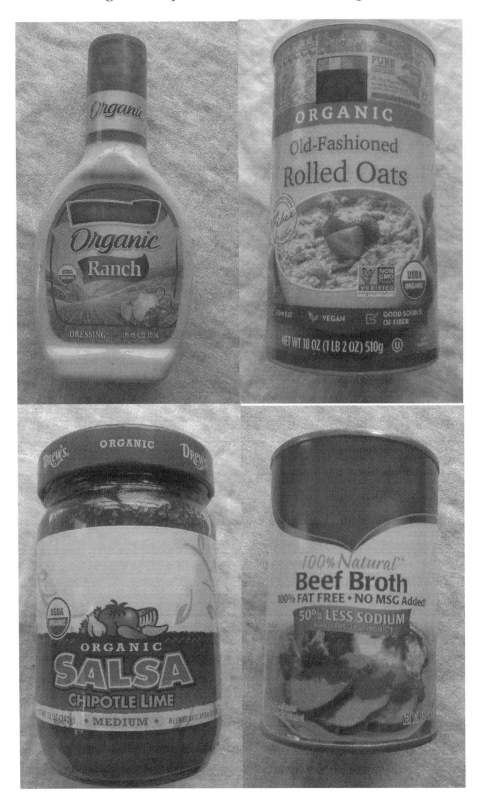

LESSON 5: SWEETENERS – SUCRALOSE

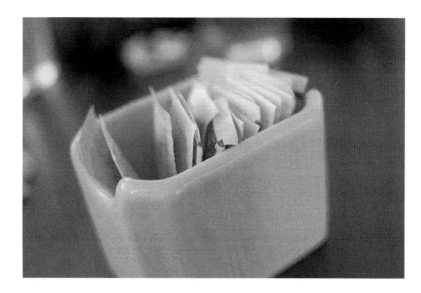

How can it *not* be a good thing? You know, sucralose, in those pretty yellow packages, being substituted for all of that bad, blood-sugar raising, teeth-rotting sugar? It turns out that this artificial sweetener could be even worse for your health than real sugar. **It was actually discovered by scientists looking for new ways to make insecticides**[1,2]. Does this sound like something healthy to you?

Making sucralose involves adding three chlorine atoms to a molecule of sucrose[2]. (Sucrose is the sugar most of us have in our kitchens for eating and baking.) So sucralose's claim that it is made from real sugar is true. However, the finished product also contains a fair amount of chlorine[1].

Chlorine is poisonous and carcinogenic, even in small amounts. (Note: Chlorine is different from Chloride, which is found naturally in sodium chloride, or NaCl, which is simple table salt. Chlorine is the stuff that keeps your swimming pool clean by killing germs.) So in the very simplest terms, sucralose is made by adding chlorine to sucrose, which is a little like adding pool chlorine to the table sugar in your kitchen.

The sucrose ends up being a chlorinated fructo-galactose molecule as the end product[1]. If that sounds complicated, it is! **The human body had long been thought unable to metabolize this substance, which is why you can consume sucralose without it affecting your calorie intake.** It is chlorinated sugar that your body can't efficiently process. However, it has now been shown that some small fraction of the sucralose ingested *is* metabolized by your body, and causes depletion of beneficial gut bacteria as a result[3,4,5,6]. In addition, sucralose puts such a stress on your body and your digestive system that one of its side effects is liver damage[3]. Sucralose has also been determined to be mutagenic, meaning that it contributes to mutations occurring in your cells, including such mutations that can result in cancer[3].

It is also important to realize that no long term human studies on the effects of sucralose have been done, and there are no independent human studies on sucralose. (meaning studies funded by someone other than the manufacturer)[6]. Research performed by the manufacturer prior to FDA approval for its use as a food additive shows numerous side effects from its consumption, but the manufacturer did not make this information public, instead only publishing the studies that show sucralose in a positive light[2].

Only 5 safety studies evaluating sucralose use by humans were reviewed by the FDA before making their decision to approve it, and the longest toxicity study involving human use of sucralose lasted only 13 weeks. **In other words, any toxic effects sucralose may have on humans consuming it long-term were not considered by the FDA**[7].

While sucralose passes through the body without much of it being metabolized, some of it is absorbed by the body, where it can cause numerous and varied side effects. One way to determine if symptoms you're having are due to sucralose is to remove it from your diet for a period of time and see if those symptoms disappear.

The most misleading statement about sucralose is that it does not contain any calories and will not affect blood sugar levels. This statement is only true about sucralose itself, and does not take into account the bulking agents used in the commercially prepared product. The sucralose mixture sold to the public also contains dextrose, sucrose, and maltodextrin, which DO count as calories and ARE capable of raising blood sugar. It follows that sucralose may not be as safe for diabetics as advertising has led them to believe[7].

Frequent consumption of non-nutritive sweeteners like sucralose is suspected to interfere with how the body regulates appetite and energy balance. Imagine how confused your metabolism will be if you eat things that taste sweet but your body does not get much of the calorie or energy boost it anticipates from those sweet-tasting foods[8]. It is thought that this mechanism is part of why the **long-term consumption of "diet" foods with artificial sweeteners often leads to increased risk of weight gain, metabolic syndrome, type 2 diabetes, and cardiovascular disease**[9].

The bags and packets available for consumer use are not pure sucralose. All artificial sweeteners use bulking agents for volume, and to make them into a useable powder, and sucralose is no different. Do you know what they use? Dextrose, sucrose, and maltodextrin, which are all various forms of.... SUGARS! A little understood truth of the sweetener industry is that all sweetener packets are at least 96 percent bulking agents, and brand-name sucralose contains 99 percent, in the form of dextrose, sucrose, and maltodextrin[7].

Sucralose can be labeled calorie free due to a loophole in the U.S. food labeling regulations. A product can be described as sugar free if a serving contains less than 5 grams of sugar, and calorie free if a serving is less than 5 calories[10]. So they set the serving size on bags at 0.5 grams and the packets contain a serving of 1 gram. One 0.5 gram serving contains 2 calories, and a one gram packet contains 4 calories. Viola! Calorie and sugar free! So there is a distinction to be made here. **Sucralose cannot raise blood sugar or contribute to your caloric intake, but the name brand form sold in stores, with its added ingredients, _can._**

The trademarked, brand-name product that is so often packaged in yellow on your store shelves can also legally be called sucralose, because it is made by replacing 3 of the -OH groups of sucrose, which is table sugar like you'd find in your kitchen, with chlorine[11]. Examine the 2 chemical structures below and show where this has occurred by circling the 3 -OH groups in sucrose that are replaced with chlorine in sucralose. *In other words, circle the areas that are different between the two drawings.*

Sucrose   **Sucralose**

True or False:

1. T / F Another name for sucralose is aspartame.

2. T / F Sucralose must not be safe for human consumption because it has not been approved by the FDA.

3. T / F Sucralose will not raise blood sugar.

4. T / F An independent study is one that has not been funded by a person or group that has a financial stake in the study's outcome.

5. T / F Sucralose passes through the human body without being absorbed at all.

Short answer question:

The two grocery store chains Whole Foods and Trader Joe's refuse to carry products containing sucralose. Imagine that you work for a store that needs to come up with a policy statement about whether or not it will sell items containing sucralose. In a few sentences, explain why your store will or will not sell sucralose.

Symptom Causes:

Here is a long list of possible side effects of sucralose. *It's important to realize that sucralose is not the only possible cause for these symptoms.* Choose 5 of these symptoms and think of at least one other cause for them. For example, anxiety could also be caused by too much caffeine, or a burning feeling on the skin could be caused by a sunburn. Fill in the spaces below based on your findings.

Possible Splenda Reaction Symptoms	
<ul><li>Flushing or redness of the skin</li><li>Burning feeling of the skin</li><li>Rash</li><li>Itching</li><li>A panicky or shaky feeling</li><li>Swelling</li><li>Blisters on the skin</li><li>Welts</li><li>Nausea</li><li>Stomach cramps</li><li>Dry heaves</li><li>Becoming withdrawn</li><li>Loss of interest in usual activities</li><li>Feeling forgetful</li><li>Moodiness</li><li>Dulled senses</li><li>Unexplained crying</li></ul>	<ul><li>Acne or acne-like rash</li><li>Anxiety</li><li>Panic attacks</li><li>Feelings of food poisoning</li><li>Headache</li><li>Seeing spots</li><li>Mental or emotional breakdown</li><li>Altered emotional state, i.e. feeling irate, impatient, hypersensitive</li><li>Pain (body, chest)</li><li>Bloated abdomen</li><li>Diarrhea</li><li>Trouble concentrating/staying in focus</li><li>Feeling depressed</li><li>Vomiting</li><li>Seizures</li><li>Shaking</li><li>Feeling faint</li></ul>

<u>Symptom</u>   <u>Other potential causes</u>

1.

2.

3.

4.

5.

ACTIVITY:
Sucralose originated during research on the development of new insecticides, and was even tested as an insecticide before its sweet taste was discovered and it began to be used as a sweetener.

Given its origin as part of insecticide research, do you think sucralose will kill ants? If you have ant hills in your yard, or some other location you notice unwanted ants, try sprinkling some sucralose nearby and come back to check for any changes. Does it kill ants? Is it an effective insecticide?

LESSON 6: SWEETENERS - ASPARTAME

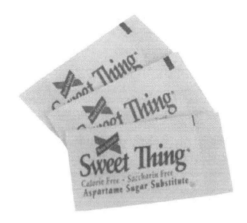

We've all heard of it, but what is aspartame? Is it healthy?

As the story goes, aspartame was discovered accidentally in 1965 when a chemist for drug company G.D. Searle spilled something in the lab as he was researching a drug for an unrelated disease. He discovered the spilled substance tasted sweet, and aspartame was born[1].

Another artificial sweetener, called cyclamate, had recently been pulled from the market, and powerful forces stood to make billions of dollars if aspartame were approved for human consumption. Searle spent many millions of dollars conducting the tests required for FDA approval, but these were not independent studies. The studies funded by Searle found no adverse effects from aspartame use, but studies funded by others did[2,3]. Through an incredible story of politics and financial manipulation, Searle won FDA approval for aspartame in 1974 through one of the most highly contested approval processes in history[1,4]. Although the controversy raged on, the FDA gave aspartame full approval as an all-purpose sweetener in 1996[1].

In 1977, the FDA initiated a criminal investigation into whether or not Searle misrepresented the results in the studies submitted during the approval process. An important point to make is that this case was never resolved. Through a series of political and legal maneuvers, the case was stalled in court until the statute of limitations expired[1]. In the meantime, and still today, aspartame continues to be sold to Americans, who consume it in diet sodas, yogurt, gelatin, pudding, multi-vitamins, and even chewing gum.

Aspartame is rapidly broken down, or hydrolyzed, in the small intestine. In fact, it is hydrolyzed so rapidly that aspartame itself never makes it into the bloodstream. Only the products of aspartame breakdown can be detected in the blood, and there are three of them: methanol, phenylalanine, and aspartic acid.

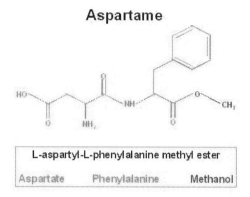

Methanol is also known as "wood alcohol", and stories abound of wood alcohol poisoning back during the days of Prohibition. Folks would destill their own spirits (think moonshine!) and if they weren't careful they could end up drinking methanol instead of the ethanol they intended to produce. That's a costly mistake, because ingestion of methanol causes serious eye problems, up to and including blindness. In addition, methanol degrades in the body to formaldehyde, which is a substance used in such things as paint remover and embalming fluid[5]. It's also a potent carcinogen and has been proven to increase the incidence of breast and prostate cancer[2].

Phenylalanine is also a product of the breakdown of aspartame. It's a naturally-occurring amino acid, which are the building blocks used to make proteins. Your body uses phenylalanine in the production of certain neurotransmitters in your brain, and these are the substances that make it possible for nerve cells to communicate with one another. Too much phenylalanine can result in stress to the brain from over-excited nerve cells, like anxiety, panic attacks, and even seizures[6]. In people who have a hereditary disease called phenylketonuria, consuming phenylalanine from aspartame can actually cause brain damage[7].

Aspartic acid (or aspartate) is also a large component of aspartame, and in lab animals it can cause similar problems, like tremors, seizures, and strokes. It serves as an "excitatory neurotransmitter" in the brain, and it can actually excite cells to death. It falls into a category of compounds known as excitotoxins, which are linked to free radical production in the body, as well as neurodegenerative diseases like Alzheimer's and Parkinson's[6].

Below are a few commonly reported symptoms of aspartame reactions. Some people may have only slight reactions, or none at all, while other people are more sensitive to it. But more people have filed complaints with the FDA for aspartame than any other substance, so clearly it poses a *potential* risk[8].

- headaches, especially migraines
- memory loss
- visual disturbances
- anxiety, nervousness
- tremors, seizures
- dizziness, loss of balance
- changes in heart rate
- nausea/vomiting/cramps/diarrhea

If you regularly consume aspartame and think your body may be sensitive to it, try cutting it out of your diet for a few weeks and note if your symptoms go away. Pregnant and lactating women should be especially cautious about aspartame because the blood-brain barrier, which prevents toxins from entering the brain, is not yet fully developed in infants and young children[9].

Supporters of aspartame claim the toxicity is minimal because of the low amounts consumed. But in addition to the reports of numerous side effects, animal tests indicate there is a cancer risk to humans who consume aspartame[11]. Is aspartame worth the risk to you?

True or False
1. T / F Aspartame is believed to contribute to cancer development.

2. T / F Seizures, headaches, and anxiety are symptoms of aspartame sensitivity.

3. T / F Cyclamate is an artificial sweetener that is a safe alternative to aspartame.

4. T / F The best way to check for aspartame toxicity is to check aspartame levels in the blood.

5. T / F Aspartame consists of aspartate, phenylalanine, and methanol.

Most of the studies on aspartame submitted to the FDA were performed by the drug company, G.D. Searle[1]. Some scientists were critical of these non-independent studies and in 1977 Jerome Bressler wrote "The Bressler Report", which claims these studies were flawed. Listed below are some of the allegations made[12]. Can you explain why these would affect the accuracy of the data obtained from the studies?

- If a lab animal died during the study, an autopsy was often delayed, sometimes by as much as one year after the animal's death.
- Tumors were removed from animals prior to health assessments of those animals being performed.

Additional material for advanced students:

Sweet Misery: A Poisoned World http://video.google.com/videoplay?docid=-6551291488524526735#

ACTIVITY:

You'll need 2 large bowls or other containers of water. (This experiment also works in the bathtub!) You will also need one can each of regular soda (containing SUGAR, not high-fructose corn syrup) and diet soda. It's best to use the same brand. For example, one can of diet Pepsi and one can of Throwback Pepsi, because it is made with real sugar. They need to be the same size.

Do you think the cans will sink or float in water? Will one sink and the other float? Why do you think this? Form a hypothesis about what you think will happen, and write it below.

Place the soda cans in water and write your observations below. Did they sink or float?

Write down your explanation for why you think this happened. Was your hypothesis proven true or false?

LESSON 7: SWEETENERS – HIGH FRUCTOSE CORN SYRUP

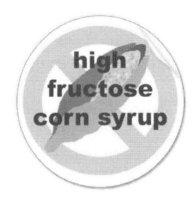

We've all heard about sugar rotting our teeth and causing weight gain. Would you be surprised to hear that these days there's rarely any sugar in soda? These days it's mostly High Fructose Corn Syrup (HFCS), and despite a multi-million dollar ad campaign from the Corn Refiners Association to convince consumers otherwise, HFCS is bad news. Check out your grocery store shelves for an increasing number of products beginning to use "No High Fructose Corn Syrup" as a selling point. The public is beginning to realize that HFCS is *not* healthy.

Genetically Modified Corn

This sweetener isn't even made from sugar; it's made from corn, the majority of which has been genetically modified. The long term effects on humans of a diet containing GMO foods are unknown because they've only been around since the 1990s. However, studies in animals conclusively show ill effects[1].

Animals fed a GMO diet have significantly decreased fertility rates, and the problem appears to worsen in successive generations. We're not just talking about lab studies on mice or rats, but farmers have reported decreased fertility in farm animals given feed containing GMO corn and soy[1]. **With the human life span being so much longer, the lifelong effects on people can't yet be measured.**

Mercury Contamination

In addition, the process by which HFCS is produced involves the use of mercury, and small amounts of mercury can remain in the finished product. Mercury is a heavy metal and is toxic even in miniscule amounts. **There is NO safe level of Mercury consumption.** Ingestion of mercury leads to nervous system damage. Even the trace amounts of mercury often present in HFCS can contribute to zinc loss, which is an essential mineral for proper brain function, and thus mercury consumption has been tied to autism and other learning disabilities in children[2,3].

But soda isn't the only thing that contains HFCS. This awful stuff is present in approximately 7 out of 10 products on your grocery store's shelves. Time to start reading labels! Here's a quote from David Wallinga, MD, of the Institute for Agriculture and Trade Policy (IATP), a co-author of two of the most significant studies on this subject.

"Mercury is toxic in all its forms. Given how much high fructose corn syrup is consumed by children, it could be a significant additional source of mercury never before considered. We are calling for immediate changes by industry and the FDA to help stop this avoidable mercury contamination of the food supply."[4]

Metabolic Effects

You may have heard that your body can't tell the difference between high fructose corn syrup and sugar. But in fact, it can. **HFCS is metabolized differently in your body than sugar, and as bad as sugar is for you, the effects of HFCS are far worse.** Fructose is the type of sugar naturally found in fruit. But HFCS is sucrose that has been altered with enzymes and chemicals to increase its sweetness. It is not found in nature, and is therefore not a natural substance. The cofactors, fiber, enzymes, and other nutrients that are present along with the fructose in fruit are not present in HFCS, which considerably alters how HFCS is metabolized, or broken down and used, by your body[5].

HFCS increases blood triglyceride levels and causes fat buildup in the liver[6]. It's also a major contributing factor to metabolic syndrome, which is a cluster of problems including inability to properly regulate blood sugar levels, obesity, high blood pressure, and heart disease, to name a few[7]. These are all health problems that used to only be seen in older people, but now are on the rise in children too. And if all that weren't bad enough, HFCS may also affect your sensitivity to appetite so you're less likely to feel full and more likely to overeat, especially when HFCS consumption is paired with a high fat diet[8]. For this and other reasons, HFCS has long been suspected to indirectly contribute to obesity[9,10].

There is one thing HFCS is good for, and that's feeding cancer cells. In laboratory studies, cancerous tumors love fructose. It seems to encourage the tumors to grow larger and spread[11,12].

As Dr. David Williams states:

"It's no wonder that cancer has moved quickly up the list of killers in our society since we started adding high-fructose corn syrup to everything from sodas to bread. With such damning and irrefutable research, I still don't understand why it hasn't become standard practice to immediately put cancer patients on fructose-free diets to help disrupt cancer growth." [13]

Deceptive Advertising and Who Pays For It?

One of the most important things to learn from this lesson is the value in researching an issue yourself before passing judgement on it. Have you ever seen the TV commercials for "corn sugar", proclaiming it to be just like sugar, and even poking fun at the controversy surrounding it? Those commercials are part of a 40 million dollar ad campaign by the Corn Refiners Association, a group of people who make HFCS. Because HFCS is cheaper than sugar and has other practical advantages in the manufacturing of processed foods, they have a vested interest in making sure sales of HFCS don't decrease[14].

A lot of money has been spent to convince the public that HFCS is safe, but in 2012 the Food and Drug Administration (FDA) denied a request from the Corn Refiners Association to label HFCS as "corn sugar", saying that sugar and HFCS are not nutritionally nor metabolically equivalent[15].

Children are taught to respect authority, and that those in charge know what's best. That's why this concept is so difficult to learn. For busy parents, it's easier to trust the opinions of those in charge too, rather than take the time to research issues ourselves. But don't trust blindly. **Keep in mind that the World Health Organization recommends a maximum consumption of 40g/day of all forms of sugar**[16]. **Remember, HFCS is not healthy, even if the FDA has approved it, and even if the stores continue to sell it.**

True or False

1. T / F HFCS is also known as corn sugar.

2. T / F HFCS causes fat to not be absorbed effectively by the digestive system.

3. T / F Almost all of the corn used to make HFCS is genetically modified.

4. T / F The mercury found in HFCS is safe because it is such a small quantity.

5. T / F The Corn Refiners Association spends lots of money to convince people to eat corn.

Study the graph below and answer the questions.

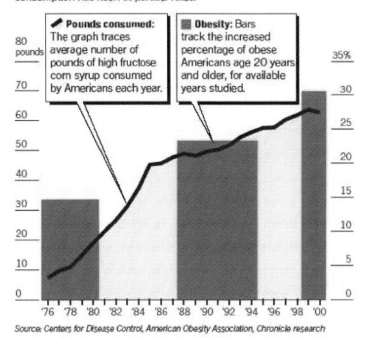

1. Between 1987 and 1994, what percentage of Americans were obese?

2. How many more Americans were obese in 1992 than in 1978? (in percent)

3. When was the largest increase in the number of pounds of HFCS consumed by Americans?
    A. 1976-1978
    B. 1978-1985
    C. 1990-1992
    D. 1999-2000

4. In 1983, how much HFCS did the average American consume?

5. What happened to HFCS consumption in 1999?

Look at this interactive map from the Centers for Disease Control. Determine the rate of obesity where you live, and for your ethnicity. http://www.cdc.gov/obesity/data/trends.html

ACTIVITY:

Although many types of food contain HFCS, most of our consumption comes from drinking soda. Below is a recipe for making your own root beer at home to reduce your consumption of HFCS from commercially prepared soda. You can try this recipe or find one of your own.

```
Recipe for Root Beer

8 cups sugar
5 gallons water (room temperature or lukewarm is best)
1 bottle root beer extract
1/2 to 1 package compressed yeast

Dissolve sugar in water. Add the root beer extract and yeast. Mix and
bottle.  Seal tightly and set in warm place. Root beer is ready for use in
10 to 12 hours. It is better if allowed to stand for several days.
```

LESSON 8: PRODUCE – FROM SEED TO TABLE

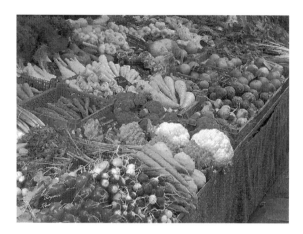

Did you know that parents' attitudes and eating habits can deeply influence what foods their kids think are healthy?[1] It's an excellent idea to explore nature together as a family and discover where foods come from! So many of us in modern society never see strawberries except in those clear plastic containers at the grocery store, and these days an autumn trip to the pumpkin patch is the closest many kids come to seeing produce growing naturally. How can you get back to nature and get in touch with *your* food?

You probably know that potatoes grow underground, but did you know sweet potato plants grow beautiful, flowering vines? Or that carrots are unusual because they don't produce seed until after their *second* growing season? If bananas only grow in tropical climates, how are they for sale in every grocery store in North America?

These days, we're so far removed from our food sources that we may not even know where some of the things we eat come from. Agriculture is a big business, and foods like pineapples and bananas are grown in one place and then shipped internationally for us to eat. Sometimes long-distance food transport occurs within the United States too, like when citrus fruits are grown in Florida, or potatoes in Idaho, and then shipped across the country to a grocery store near you.

Food must be grown in the right climate and with proper soil and other conditions, and each fruit or vegetable's requirements are a little different. Potatoes may not grow as well in Mississippi, for example, as they do in Idaho, and grapefruit doesn't grow well in New Hampshire at all. So transportation of food is necessary in order to enjoy out-of-season produce year round, or in areas where it's impossible to grow some things locally.

Produce is transported in trucks, on trains, and sometimes even aboard ships. **Food miles** is a term measuring the distance between where food was grown, and where it ends up on the grocery store shelf[2]. In the winter when much of the U.S. has weather too cold for growing, a fair amount of our produce is shipped here from farms in Mexico and South America, where warm weather that time of year makes farming profitable.

Have you ever heard the slogan **"Eat Local"**? Some people may be concerned about greenhouse gas emissions from the transport of food long distances, which can be avoided by only buying foods grown in your local area. Other people may want to support the local economy by promoting local foods over foods brought in from far away. Eating locally grown food helps to build a sense of community among farmers and their customers, people like....YOU! Plus, food grown locally tends to be fresher when you eat it, and therefore more nutritious than foods that were harvested many days ago and shipped to you.

In the United States, the top food crops grown are corn, soybeans, and wheat. The U.S. grows more than 80% of the world's corn. Much of it is used as livestock feed, and the rest is used in food sources for people, like corn chips and high fructose corn syrup. Corn also has industrial uses, like in the production of ethanol to use as fuel for cars. Soybeans grown in the U.S. account for about half of world production, and our wheat production is 13% of the wheat grown in the entire world[3].

Given that corn and soybeans are the most plentiful crops in the U.S. and both are typically harvested in October, that's a busy time of year for farmers, second only to the spring planting season. Most field crops are harvested by huge agricultural machines like combines, but most fruits and other smaller food crops are still harvested by hand. Once harvested, the trip to market begins!

What Food Miles Can Tell You:

- How far away your food came from.

- How much energy was used to transport your food to you.

- How much pollution was generated by that transport.

- How fresh your food might be.

- How connected you are, economically and socially, to regional farmers.

- Where the lands are that your stomach is walking on.

What Food Miles Can't Tell You:

- How much energy was used in growing and packaging your food.

- How ecologically-sustainable the practices of the farmers were.

- How nutritious your food is (although the time and packaging needed for extensive transport might have some effect).

- How much energy you used to go shopping and to prepare your food.

- How important your purchases are to the well-being of farmers in other parts of the world.

(The graphic above is used with permission of the Farmscape Ecology Program at Hawthorne Valley Farm.)[4]

QUESTIONS:

1. Can you get some idea of how fresh your food might be, based upon its food miles?

2. If you know the food miles of your food, can you tell how much energy was used to grow the food?

3. List at least 3 reasons people might want to "eat local".

4. Can food miles tell you if your produce was grown organically?

5. What are some ways foods are transported from where they are grown to the stores where they are sold?

6. Explain why potatoes don't grow well in Mississippi and grapefruit doesn't grow well in New Hampshire.

7. Would it be better to harvest a crop of strawberries with large farm equipment, or to pick them by hand? Why?

8. What is the number one crop grown in the U.S?

9. What crop is ethanol made from?

10. In what month are most crops, especially corn and soybeans, harvested?

DISCUSSION QUESTION:

If you were a farmer, would you prefer to sell your produce at local markets, or have it shipped across the country to be sold? Explain your answer. Some things to consider are how much demand there is for your product, and how much money you could earn from each of the options.

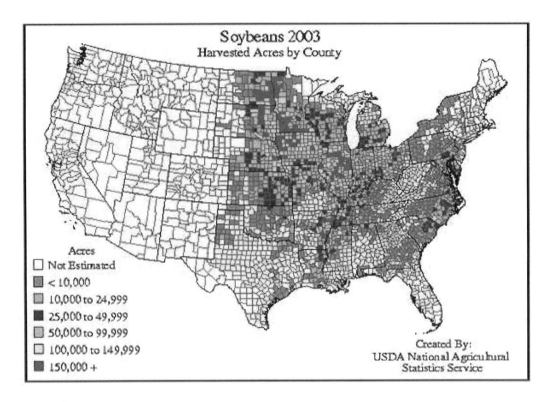

Look at the map above. Where are the most soybeans grown? The least? Do you think soybeans grow well in hot, dry climates?

ADDITIONAL RESEARCH TOPICS:
1. What is sorghum, and how much is grown in the U.S?

2. Find out what crops are most commonly grown where you live.

ACTIVITIES:
Check out the website www.foodmiles.com for an interactive calculator you can use to figure out how many miles your food has traveled before it reaches you.

Head to the store and see if you can find produce shipped in from other countries. (Hint: The labels on bananas are a great first place to look!)

LESSON 9: PRODUCE – BASIC BOTANY OF EDIBLE PLANTS

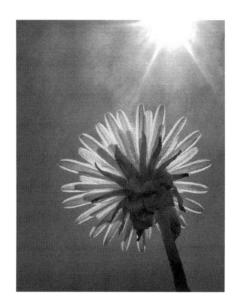

Botany is the study of plants, but we're going to focus our nutrition study specifically on the botany of edible plants. People can eat many parts of plants, such as the stems, like celery, the leaves, like lettuce, and the seeds, like sunflower seeds. The roots and fruits of many plants are also edible. Did you know that the tomatoes we eat are actually the fruit of the tomato plant? Or that carrots are roots that grow underground?

Kids who get their hands dirty and learn to garden are more likely to eat healthier diets and to try new and different fruits and vegetables[1,2]. Besides the health benefits, it's a lot of fun to watch something grow, *and eat it*, if you planted and cared for it yourself. So let's learn about the plants we eat!

Functions of the Different Parts of Plants

Each part of a plant has its own function, and the parts must all work together to keep the plant healthy.

ROOTS - absorb water from the soil
STEM - transports water from the roots to the leaves
LEAVES - this is where photosynthesis occurs
FLOWER - not all plants have flowers, but for those that do, the flower is where pollination occurs

SEEDS - germinate and grow to produce new plants

Animals are **heterotrophic**, which means they must eat to survive. Plants are **autotrophic**, meaning they can produce their own food, rather than having to eat it. They do this through a process called **photosynthesis**.

Edible Wild Plants

You produce doesn't have to be cultivated on a farm! Discovering the many uses of dandelions is a fun way to introduce the concept that wild foods can be edible.

Dandelion cookies, anyone? Kids: you can help by picking dandelions, then learning how to pull the petals off by holding the green flower base firmly with one hand and pulling the yellow parts off as a group with the other hand. Wash them with clean water and pat them dry. Now you're ready to make dandelion cookies!

DANDELION FLOWER COOKIES
1/2 cup oil
1/2 cup honey
2 eggs
1 teaspoon almond extract
1 cup all-purpose flour
1 cup rolled oats
1/2 cup dandelion florets

Combine oil and honey and beat in the two eggs and almond extract. Stir in flour, oatmeal and washed dandelion florets. Add teaspoonfuls of batter to a lightly greased cookie sheet. Bake at 375 degrees for about 12 minutes.

IMPORTANT: Dandelions are only one type of edible wild plant. All parts of the dandelion plant are edible, not just the flowers. Some other edible plants are nettles and garlic mustard[3]. **If you plan to begin eating wild plants, it's a good idea to familiarize yourself with all of the poisonous plants in your area first.** Be very careful, because they can sometimes be hard to identify. Have an adult help!

Poisonous Plants

Although many parts of some plants are edible, it's important to note that many other plants cannot safely be eaten. Many poisonous plants exist too, so make sure you know the difference! Poison ivy, poison oak, and poison sumac are three of the most widely known poisonous plants, but they're poisonous to touch. Most people wouldn't even think of eating them!

Some plants have edible parts, and poisonous parts too. The root of the potato plant is safe to eat. It's a potato! But any part of this plant growing above ground, like the leaves and stem, is toxic[4]. The stems of a rhubarb plant are edible, but the leaves are poisonous[5]. Can you think of any other examples?

Most people wouldn't know how to recognize hemlock, but the ancient Greek philosopher Socrates ate some to commit suicide![6] **A good rule of thumb is to assume you shouldn't eat any unidentified plant, unless a parent says it's safe.**

ACTIVITY:
Make a booklet out of paper, in any style you wish, but with the pages labeled as follows:

    Roots   Leaves
    Stems   Fruits
    Flowers Seeds

Collect several grocery store ads, and cut out pictures of produce. You can also search for pictures online, or draw them yourself. Paste the pictures onto the correct page to show what part of that plant people eat. For example, lettuce would go on the "leaves" page.

QUESTIONS:

1. Where in a plant does photosynthesis occur?

2. What is the function of the roots?

3. What does autotrophic mean?

4. Name one plant, which was discussed in this lesson, where ALL of its parts are edible.

5. If you aren't sure if a particular wild plant is edible or poisonous, what should you do?

PROJECT:
Listed below are several unusual plants that are edible but not as common as what you probably eat on an everyday basis. Have you heard of any of them? Have you eaten any of them?

Choose one and spend some time researching it. Prepare a report on your plant, explaining what it looks like, where and how it is grown, how it is eaten, what it tastes like, etc. Present the report to your family to share what you have learned. (Optional: See if you can find your chosen food at the store so you can buy some to sample!)

quince	mangosteen	watercress	passion fruit
loquat	salsify	cassava	jackfruit
starfruit	bok choy	parsnip	tamarillo
rutabaga	jicama	leek	gooseberries
guava	kohlrabi	filbert	pawpaw

OPTIONAL - FOR ADDITIONAL READING:

"Dandelions: Not the nuisance weed you always thought" by Marie Hoyer
http://www.theprairiestar.com/entertainment/columnists/recipes_and_reflections/dandelions-not-the-nuisance-weed-you-always-thought/article_9d94b662-8c96-11e0-a29c-001cc4c03286.html

"How to Become a Botanist"
http://www.ehow.com/video_4872712_become-botanist.html

"Meet the Plant Parts"
This is an interactive game to help kids learn what plant part their favorite vegetables are, and they do this by building a salad with their correct answers!
http://www.hhmi.org/coolscience/forkids/vegquiz/plantparts.html

Identification of edible and poisonous plants
http://www.safekid.org/plants.htm

LESSON 10: SUSTAINABLE FARMING

Examine the two pictures of cattle below. The photo on the left is a confined feeding operation, and the photo on the right shows rotational grazing.

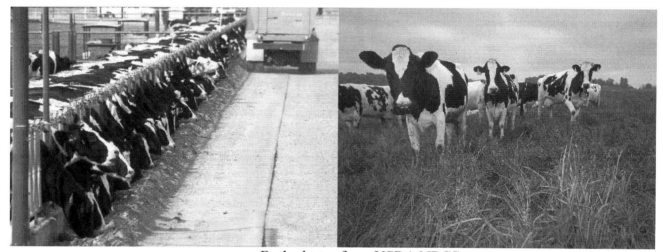

Both photos from USDA NRCS.

What are some of the differences in how these cows are being fed? Are there any similarities? Which cows do you think are healthier? Is one or the other method of feeding better for the land? Can you guess which method employs sustainable farming practices?

Many people today are disconnected from the growing of the food they eat. We learn to think of food production as a one-sided affair: how to grow the best crop or get livestock raised and to the market as quickly as possible[1]. But the opposite perspective is important too. How does our food production affect the environment and the rest of the world around us?

Sustainable farming is a large category of agricultural practices that promote responsible use of land and natural resources and promote a high quality of life for farmers and farming communities. The exact definition sometimes depends on who you ask. But generally, sustainable farming results in healthier livestock and produce, is better for the earth than conventional farming, and allows small farmers, rather than large agri-businesses, to thrive.

Sustainable farmers may avoid pesticides and herbicides which could harm bees needed for pollination of crops. They may preserve bee habitats and make their land a place bees would like to visit. They may choose to raise their livestock without the routine use of antibiotics[2]. **They may also try to preserve the ecology and maintain the biodiversity of the land.** You can do this in your own backyard by using hummingbird feeders, providing bird houses, and growing plants that butterflies enjoy, in order to encourage pollinators and other wildlife to remain in the area.

Soil in different areas will contain different amounts of minerals that plants need to grow, such as phosphorus, calcium, magnesium, nitrogen, and potassium. Rather than adding chemical fertilizers to the soil to increase the amount of these minerals present, **sustainable farmers might use natural methods to add important nutrients to the soil.** Composting is one way you can do this yourself, by collecting yard waste and kitchen scraps and letting them decompose in a compost bin or compost pile in your yard. When compost is added to the soil, it increases the levels of valuable nutrients that plants need to thrive.

Sustainable farmers often use something called crop rotation. This means they change which crops they grow in which fields each year. Different crops deplete different nutrients from the soil, so if a farmer grew corn in the same field every year, that soil would be very deficient in the nutrients corn plants need a lot. Rotating the crops helps prevent this.

Farmers may even choose to leave a field fallow for a season, which means to not grow anything at all there, to give the soil a chance to recover. They could also plant cover crops in certain fields. **Cover crops are non-cash crops, only grown to replace some of the nutrients in the soil, not to be sold for profit.** Alfalfa and many types of beans are often grown as cover crops. Rather than being harvested, they are plowed under, to help increase the nitrogen level in the soil. Sometimes these types of cover crops are referred to as "green manure" because they're a natural fertilizer, just like compost would be.

The rotational grazing system can also help break pest cycles, and this is significant since most **sustainable farmers try not to use chemical insecticides**. Sometimes, a cover crop will be planted nearby because it provides a favorable habitat of a certain type of pest. The pests will move to the field with the cover crop, and leave the main crop alone. Or the cover crop could encourage growth of a natural predator to the insects affecting the main crop, thus protecting the main crop naturally.

Companion planting can be used to help avoid the need for chemical pesticides too. Some plants can be beneficial to others. For example, marigold flowers help deter insect pests near tomatoes. Planting garlic near your vegetables can prevent Japanese beetles from devouring your crop. There are countless other examples of these combinations. Companion planting is especially useful to organic farmers who don't use chemicals, but still need ways to control pests.

Even the design of the farm can help. For example, the practice of "strip cropping" helps to **reduce wind and water erosion of the soil**. Crops are planted in alternating strips either at right angles or following the contour of the land. This is just one example of the conservation efforts sustainable farmers practice.

Sustainable farmers strive to be good stewards of the land. They want to take care of the land so it will continue to produce for them. They take care of their livestock too, by keeping them healthy and feeding them what nature intended for them to eat. Cows were not designed to eat corn and although labels in your grocery store's meat department tout "grain-fed" as a buying point, it isn't. Cows were meant to graze on grass, not eat corn and the assorted other foodstuffs they are fed on factory farms to get them to slaughter weight more quickly. Cows are much healthier when they eat grass, and their meat is healthier for people to eat when they are grass-fed, too.

Sustainable farmers are often organic farmers. Although there is a lot of overlap between the practices of organic farmers and sustainable farmers, it is more important to make the distinction between these types of farming and the big agri-business farming. **Large corporations control much of the farmland in this country, and they use whatever means necessary to make their businesses profitable.** The quality of the food produced suffers, as does the condition of the land they're farming, because sometimes neither is properly cared for. Much can be learned when local farmers are respected for their traditions and the wisdom they've gained over the years refining their sustainable practices[3].

Sustainable farming means caring for the land and protecting natural habitats and wildlife as much as possible. It means conserving nature's resources and avoiding chemicals to boost production, and it also means supporting local, small farms so they can compete against the larger factory farm operations. Sustainable farming affects nutrition because people who value these types of practices, like eating locally grown food and minimizing the use of chemicals, tend to eat better and be healthier[4].

WRITING:
Thinking back to the pictures at the beginning, if you were a cattle farmer, which feeding method would you prefer to use? Explain why, and remember to include some of the details from the discussion above in your answer.

Short answer questions:
1. What is green manure?

2. Why would a farmer want to preserve the habitat of bees, wild birds, and butterflies?

3. What are some of the minerals in soil that plants need to grow?

4. What does it mean to be a good steward of the land?

5. What is something you could do in your own backyard garden to practice sustainable farming methods?

True or False:

1. T F Cows are often fed grain because it is better for them than eating grass.

2. T F   Plutonium is an important mineral in soil that helps plants thrive.

3. T F   Alfalfa is one type of cover crop that is often plowed under, rather than sold for profit.

4. T F   Strip cropping means to strip away the topsoil before planting.

5. T F   An insecticide kills unwanted weeds.

Optional - Sources for Additional Information:

National Sustainable Agriculture Coalition http://sustainableagriculture.net/blog/farmers-seek-justice-in-the-heartland/

Find a farmers market near you
http://www.localharvest.org/

The Well-Fed Homestead blog
"Teaching Kids About Sustainable Agriculture" http://www.wellfedhomestead.com/2011/01/31/teaching-kids-about-sustainable-agriculture/

PROJECT: Grow a "Three Sisters" Garden

Some Native American Indians practiced this form of gardening by planting 3 types of seeds into a single hole in a mound of dirt. They planted corn, squash, and pole beans. The 3 plants form an ecosystem where they depend on one another. The tall corn plants provide shade to the beans and squash, and the pole beans are able to grow up the tall corn plants like a trellis.   The beans have a type of bacteria on their roots that absorb nitrogen from the air and "fixes" it into useable form, thereby enriching the soil for other crops. The squash plants have large, prickly leaves that protect the beans and corn from predators and keep weeds from growing[6]. This is a simple example of companion planting, and if your family has a backyard garden, you could even try planting this yourself!

Based on the description, draw a picture of what you think a Three Sisters Garden would look like.

LESSON 11: GRASS-FED AND PASTURED MEATS

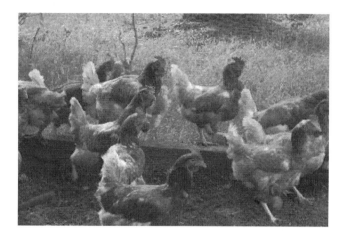

Have you seen labels on packages of meat in the store that say "grain-fed" or "pasture-raised"? Why does it matter what your meat eats? Don't chickens prefer to eat chicken feed, rather than having to wander about searching for grass and bugs to eat? Beef is beef, right? Wrong!

NUTRITIONAL DIFFERENCES

Meat from grass-fed animals is lower in fat, and since fat is very high in calories, this means you can eat a grass-fed steak and consume fewer calories than if you ate the same size steak from a grain-fed animal. Not only that, but the composition of the fat differs too. **Grass-fed animals contain much higher amounts of Omega-3 fats**, which are much healthier. Grain-fed animals contain more Omega-6 fats[1,2].

While we do need some Omega-6 fat in our diet, we need much more Omega-3, and eating grain-fed meat tends to throw the ratio of Omega-3 and Omega-6 fats in your body way off. Omega-3 fats help prevent cancer, and they have very positive effects on the heart and circulatory system. Omega-3 fats are important to other body systems, too. People who have plenty of Omega-3 in their system have a lower risk of heart attack and cancer, and lower incidence of things like Alzheimer's disease, schizophrenia, attention-deficit disorder, high blood pressure, and many others[3].

Animals raised on pasture have significantly higher levels of Conjugated Linoleic Acids, or CLAs, than their grain-fed counterparts. The particular type of CLA found in meat and dairy products is a potent cancer fighter. Studies have shown that people who regularly consume grass-fed and pastured meats and dairy products have a lower rate of cancer[4].

FACTORY-FARM FEEDING PRACTICES

Cows aren't meant to eat chocolate and other candy either, but some large livestock operations save money on feed by filling the animals' bellies with the leftovers and rejects from factories that churn out processed food. The practice is so prevalent that one study, in particular, came out with recommended levels of 5 pounds of candy and 2 pounds of chocolate per day, for each cow. Cows are also commonly fed mixtures of other by-products like unwanted orange peels from orange juice production, and seeds from cotton plants when the cotton fibers are harvested to make fabric[5]. None of this is what a cow's body was designed to eat. Can you imagine a cow actually *choosing* to eat these things? No, if cows had a say in the matter, they would choose to roam the pasture and eat grass, not eat gummy bears and orange peels!

MEAT LABELS

Is "vegetarian-fed" meat the same as grass-fed or pastured? NO. Vegetarian-fed animals are not necessarily given grass or pasture. They are much more likely to have been fed grains like corn[6]. **Watch the labels closely, because "vegetarian-fed" is not as good as it sounds!**

How about a meat label that says "natural"? Actually, the term "natural" is not regulated and has no fixed definition, so "natural" can mean anything the food producer wants it to[6]. Don't count on "natural" meats being any healthier!

IN THE NEWS...

Read this article published by a local TV news station in Kentucky. What do you think of this farmer's approach to animal nutrition? Would you make the same decision that he did?

Cows eating candy during the drought

Published : Thursday, 16 Aug 2012, 7:53 AM EDT

MAYFIELD, Ky. (CNN/WPSD) - Ranchers have struggled with skyrocketing corn prices, because the drought has made feeding their livestock very expensive. But one rancher has turned to a very sweet solution.

At Mayfield's United Livestock Commodities, owner Joseph Watson is tweaking the recipe for success.

"Just to be able to survive, we have to look for other sources of nutrition," he said.

His 1,400 cattle are no longer feeding off corn. The prices, Watson says, are too high to keep corn in stock. So earlier this year, he began to buy second-hand candy.

"It has a higher ratio of fat than actually feeding straight corn," Watson explained. "It's hard to believe it will work but we've already seen the results of it now."

Watson mixes the candy with an ethanol by-product and a mineral nutrient. He says the cows have not shown any health problems from eating the candy, and they are gaining weight as they should.

"This ration is balanced to have not too much fat in it," he said.

The packaged candy comes from various companies at a discounted rate because it is not fit for store shelves.

"Salvage is a problem for a lot of these companies and they're proud to have a place to go with it," said Watson.

FAIR USE: http://www.wpri.com/dpps/entertainment/must_see_video/cows-eating-candy-during-the-drought-nd12-jgr_4323303 Alternate link: https://www.youtube.com/watch?v=WoKksgAA8lE

TRUE OR FALSE:

1. T F   Grass-fed meat contains a higher percentage of Omega-3 fats than grain-fed meats do.

2. T F   Chickens prefer to eat bagged chicken-feed rather than having to search for their own grass and bugs in a pasture or yard.

3. T F   Omega-6 fats are not necessary for human health.

4. T F   CLA stands for carbonated living acid.

5. T F   Raising chickens and cows on pasture is part of the concept of sustainable farming.

SHORT ANSWER QUESTIONS:
Look back through the lesson to find the answers to these questions.

1. What did nature intend for chickens to eat? How about cows?

2. Explain why a grass-fed steak has fewer calories than a grain-fed steak of the same size.

MULTIPLE CHOICE:

1. If a package of meat in the store is labeled "vegetarian-fed", what did the animal likely eat?
    A. vegetables
    B. corn
    C. grass
    D. hay
    E. any of the above

2. Which nutrients in grass-fed beef are responsible for people having a lower risk of cancer?

A. Omega-3 fats and CLAs
B. Omega-6 fats and CLAs
C. CLAs only
D. canola oil

3. By-product foodstuffs fed to cows may contain which of the following?
    A. orange peels
    B. cotton seeds
    C. chocolate
    D. parts of the corn plant other than the corn kernels
    E. all of the above

4. What did mother nature intend for chickens to eat?
    A. gummy bears
    B. bugs
    C. grass and weeds
    D. grains like corn
    E. both B and C are correct

5. Why would a farmer want to feed his animals things other than what they were naturally designed to eat?

    A. he knows better than mother nature
    B. he thinks the animals like the taste of these other foods better
    C. he can save money this way and earn a greater profit
    D. he doesn't want food to go to waste, so he feeds the byproduct foodstuffs to his livestock

ACTIVITY:
The next time you're at the grocery store, take a look in the meat department and see if you can find labels on the packages for grain-fed beef, grass-fed beef, and pastured poultry. Note how the "grain-fed" beef is touted as a selling point to consumers, even though it is far less healthy for them to eat.

FOR ADVANCED STUDENTS:
There are many more health advantages to grass-fed and pastured meats than what was covered in this lesson. Explore the following website, and make a list of the benefits you learn about.
http://www.eatwild.com/healthbenefits.htm

OTHER RESOURCES: There's a great resource on YouTube called "Dairy Cow Nutrition: What Does a Cow Eat?" You can search You Tube for it by title, or try this link:
http://youtu.be/xZ9G2LOkxVg

Want to find local pastured poultry or grass-fed beef? Search http://eatwild.com/.

LESSON 12: LIFE CYCLES AND ANIMAL HUSBANDRY BASICS

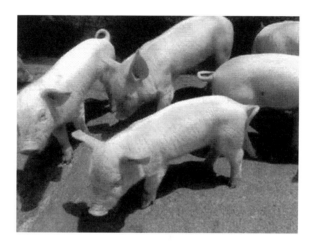

Animal husbandry is the science of breeding and raising livestock, often for food. Some of the more common domestic animals raised for food are cows, pigs, and chickens. Some animals are raised for other uses too, like sheep raised for their wool.

But your stereotypical "Old MacDonald" type of farmer isn't the only one to be skilled in the principles of animal husbandry, or raising and caring for livestock. Cowboys of the old west were part of this practice too, since they took part in cattle drives and played a large role in caring for cows that were being raised as food. Shepherds fulfill a similar role with sheep and goats. It takes a refined skill set to raise fish for human consumption, too. As you can see, animal husbandry encompasses many things. In its broadest sense, animal husbandry includes caring for an animal's biological, physiological, and social needs. It also includes breeding animals to emphasize desirable traits.

With so many big food production corporations and large-scale farms here in the U.S., the details of animal husbandry are often left to executives with college degrees in agriculture and farming. But these principles are vitally important on smaller farms and in developing countries who do not yet have a strong agricultural framework. In some places, teaching people how to farm and raise livestock could make a big difference in eliminating hunger[1]. Here in this country, formal agricultural education programs like Future Farmers of America teach young people the basics of farming[2]. The 4H program also provides programming and apprenticeships for kids who want to learn more about farming and livestock[3].

The most high quality finished products come from healthy, happy animals. Caring for an animal's welfare includes it's nutrition, reproduction, and behavior. Knowing how a particular species reproduces can help with making sure mates are available during fertile periods. In some animals, artificial insemination is often practiced, which replaces normal mating practices with a more scientific process, ensuring the male and female gametes join at the appropriate time.

Animal husbandry also includes making sure animals raised for food do not become too crowded due to overpopulation. Farmers must determine their **population status** and predict future population status, in order to plan for the needs of their animals. For example, if a farmer has 10 pigs, he needs to consider how many of these pigs are likely to breed and produce offspring that he would also need to care for. Does his farm have enough space for more pigs? Enough food, and a reliable fresh water source for more pigs? Once he evaluates the situation, he can plan accordingly.

It's important to understand the life cycles of animals in your care. How long is the typical life span, and at what age can the animals be bred, and what age are they ready for market? Some animals grow faster than others. A meat chicken may be ready for market in just a few months, but another breed of chicken that is being raised for laying eggs, may not lay its first egg until it is many months old.

TRUE OR FALSE:
1. T / F   Livestock are not always raised for food. There are other products we get from animals too.

2. T / F   Cowboys have participated in animal husbandry.

3. T / F   Different breeds of chicken are raised for meat or for laying eggs, depending on what that breed is best at.

4. T / F   Caring for an animal's welfare includes it's nutrition, reproduction, and behavior.

5. T / F   A fish farmer doesn't need to pay attention to the population status of his fish.

ACTIVITY: Visit a farm in person! If you know someone who raises animals, you could probably learn a lot from them, or you could take a field trip to a local farm that's open to the public. Another option is to use the internet to learn more - Try exploring the website of the Snayfwickby Farm (http://home.freeuk.net/elloughton13/sfarm.htm) to learn more about farm life.

CRITICAL THINKING: Pretend you work at a large zoo, and your job is to plan a way to breed the zoo's amur leopard. You know that in the wild, the male can often seriously injure the female during mating, and you'd rather not have the zoo's leopard harmed. There are no male amur leopards available at your zoo, although a few are present at other zoos, and in the wild. Devise a way to ensure breeding of this female leopard, and explain your plan below.

The farmer at a cattle ranch needs to breed his female cows but he knows that in the past his bulls have all produced offspring with suboptimal characteristics. He really wants to improve the quality of his livestock.

His options include buying new bulls to impregnate his female cows, or arranging for a bull from the neighboring ranch to father this next round of calves. Which do you think is a better choice? Why?

Imagine that your pig farm has 50 pigs and in recent years, an average of 10 new pigs are born each spring. Your current expenditure to feed and care for your pigs is $200/month, and the pigs sell for $100 each at market when they're 6 months old. Answer the following questions:

1. How many pigs will you have by summer, assuming none are sold at market between now and then?

2. How much will your monthly costs be for your pigs this summer?

3. If you plan to sell 10 of your adult pigs at the market in the fall, how much could you get for them?

4. What does it cost to raise each piglet for 6 months, until they can be sold?

5. Based upon your answer to #4, how much profit are you making on each pig sold at the market for $100?

FARM CAREERS:
Read the information from the BLS Occupational Outlook Handbook about careers working with animals, particularly on farms. Then explain whether or not you would enjoy one of these jobs. Give several supporting details to explain your position.
http://www.bls.gov/ooh/Farming-Fishing-and-Forestry/Agricultural-workers.htm

LESSON 13: DAIRY - WHAT IS PASTEURIZATION?

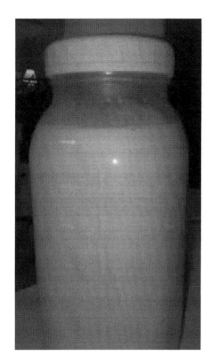

Pasteurization is a process that uses heat to kill microorganisms in food. This is most commonly used for milk and other dairy products, but can be applied to certain other foods as well. **The key point to remember about pasteurization is that it is not selective as to which microorganisms it kills, and it kills almost everything present in the product.**

There's a lot of controversy these days about pasteurization, over this very point. Some people think it's best to not allow ANY microorganisms in their food, but there are some bacteria, for example, that are beneficial. It's safe, and even desirable, to consume these beneficial bacteria. You do this every time you eat yogurt!

You may not know it, but there are millions of bacteria living in your intestines right now. Our bodies are home to these beneficial bacteria because they help us digest food, keep the harmful bacteria in check, and even aid our immune systems to keep us healthy. When you drink pasteurized milk, you are keeping the harmful bacteria from entering your body, but you are also keep beneficial bacteria, enzymes, and other nutrients out as well[1,2,5].

The process of pasteurization was invented by a chemist in France named **Louis Pasteur**. He discovered that heating milk killed the germs in it that could sometimes make people sick. This was back in the 1800s, and long before anyone knew that some of the bacteria in milk were actually good for us, so at this point in history, pasteurization was an incredible new development. Pasteurizing milk reduced the transmission of disease-causing microorganisms to humans, and far fewer people got sick[3].

In fact, here in the United States, the federal government requires any milk for human consumption to be pasteurized. The law states that **milk must be heated to 161.5 degrees for a minimum of 15 seconds**. There's a trade-off though, because heating the milk like this does compromise the taste. Pasteurized milk does taste a little different than raw milk. Pasteurizing in this way attempts to kill *most* of the microorganisms while also changing the taste as little as possible[4].

There's another method of pasteurization, called **ultra-high temperature pasteurization, or UHT**, which kills *all* of the microorganisms in the milk, making it completely sterile. The milk is heated to 285 degrees for 1-2 seconds. This unmistakably does change the taste of the milk, but some people prefer to kill all the microorganisms, believing this milk is safer to consume. If you've ever seen milk packaged in boxes, similar to how juice boxes are packaged, this form of shelf-stable milk has been treated by UHT pasteurization[4].

Have you ever seen milk with a layer of cream that has risen to the surface? Milk contains quite a bit of fat, or cream, which is lighter than the liquid milk and will rise to the top. The layer of cream on the top can be skimmed off and used to make butter, leaving behind the skimmed milk. Look at the picture of milk on the previous page and see if you can find the line between the cream and milk.

When the milk is cooled after being pasteurized, it is usually homogenized, or mixed up, so people drinking it don't need to skim the cream off. This step is not required by law, but most milk producers do homogenize their milk. **Homogenization is the process of mixing the milk**, or more specifically, breaking the fat globules into such small particles that they do not separate back into cream, but remain in solution. Some health food stores or gourmet shops do carry non-homogenized milk, and it might be fun for your family to try some. You can observe the layer of cream at the top, skim it off, and even make butter from it!

Raw milk is simply milk straight from the cow, not pasteurized at all. If you're interested in learning more about the health benefits of drinking raw milk, the Weston A. Price Foundation (http://www.westonaprice.org/) is a good place to start.

There are legal methods for buying raw milk for your family to drink, but it is important to understand the laws and follow them. There have been some well-publicized cases recently of FDA officials raiding farms who sell raw milk outside of the law, and accusations from farmers of government officials using intimidation tactics to get them to stop selling raw milk[6]. On the other hand, raw milk is considered safe enough that citizens in Italy and some other European countries can buy it in vending machines![7]

Regardless of your stance on this matter, it's important to understand that dairy farmers in big agri-business stand to lose a lot of money if raw milk becomes popular. Make sure you research both sides of the raw milk issue before deciding what you believe is the truth.

ACTIVITY:
Check the expiration dates on the milk in the grocery store. Many people think that organic milk is much healthier, but check the expiration dates of the various types of milk available. You may notice that some of the containers of milk have expiration dates much further out than the others. Read the labels more closely, and you'll see that much of the milk on store shelves is now UHT pasteurized. **Making the milk completely sterile is the only way to achieve such a long shelf-life.** You should decide for yourself if UHT milk (organic or not) is something you want to drink. Milk producers may prefer this because the longer shelf-life means higher profits, although not necessarily a healthier product for the consumer.

TRUE OR FALSE

1. T / F The cream can easily be skimmed off the top of homogenized milk.

2. T / F Louis Pasteur invented the process of homogenization.

3. T / F While the federal government in the United States requires all milk for human consumption to be pasteurized, there are some legal means for obtaining raw milk for your family to drink.

4. T / F The abbreviation UHT stands for "under high temperature", which is a technique for pasteurizing milk.

5. T / F Most people agree that pasteurization alters the taste of milk.

SHORT ANSWER:

1. Describe the difference between pasteurization and UHT pasteurization.

2. What are beneficial bacteria?

CRITICAL THINKING

Below is an advertisement for a "cream separator", which was published in the early 1900s. Knowing that cream is lighter in weight than milk, how do you think this device worked?

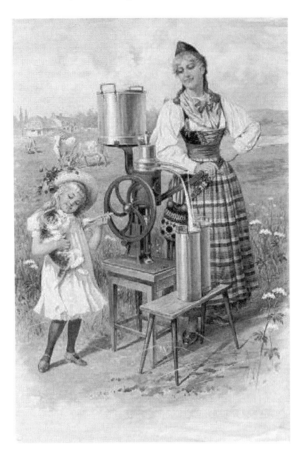

Additional Resources:

There's a video to teach kids about pasteurization over at the Brain Pop website. (This is a paid site, but parents can sign up for a free trial.)
http://www.brainpop.com/technology/healthandsafety/pasteurization/preview.weml

There's a song about raw milk and the fight to legalize it that you can listen to here: The Raw Milk Song
http://www.letslegalizeit.com/

Wondering where to buy raw milk near you? Try this site: http://www.realmilk.com/where1.html

LESSON 14: DAIRY - CHEESE, BUTTER, MILK, CURDS & WHEY, BUTTERMILK, YOGURT

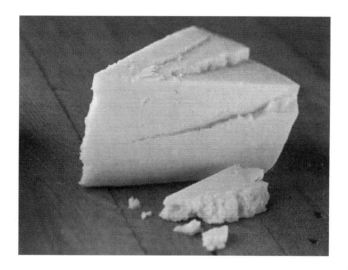

What do cheese, butter, curds & whey, buttermilk, and yogurt have in common? They're all made from milk! This means they're all part of the dairy food group, and they're all excellent sources of calcium, which your body needs for strong bones.

Whipped cream
As we learned in the previous lesson, when milk is not homogenized, or mixed up, the cream will rise to the top, where it can be skimmed off. If you whip the cream enough, it will become whipped cream[1]. (Not like the "whipped topping" you find in the grocery store in plastic tubs, and not like the stuff the comes in a can, either!) Real whipped cream is a fine and tasty treat to put on desserts!

Butter and Buttermilk
However, if you continue whipping the cream, past the point where whipped cream is formed, it will actually become butter. Butter is an accumulation of the fat present in milk. When the butter forms as a solid substance, there will be a little bit of liquid leftover, which is called buttermilk. This buttermilk has a bit of a sour taste to it, and despite its name, contains very little butter. (There may be a few specks of butter left in the buttermilk if you weren't able to effectively remove it all.) You can think of buttermilk as the milk that is leftover after making butter[1].

ACTIVITY: There's no better way to understand this process than to try it in your own kitchen! If you can find non-homogenized milk, that would be the best starting point because you can skim the cream off yourself. Otherwise, you could buy some whipping cream and use your mixer on high speed to transform it into whipped cream, then butter and buttermilk.

These days, most buttermilk you buy in a store isn't true buttermilk at all. It's usually milk that has a particular type of bacteria added to it, which allows it to begin the fermentation process. A bit of fermentation gives the milk the traditional slightly sour taste of buttermilk. This product is sold as "cultured buttermilk".[1] Most of the time, if you want *real* buttermilk, you'll have to make it yourself.

Cheese
To make cheese, an enzyme called rennet is added to milk. This causes the milk to curdle, or form curds. The liquid left over when the curds form is called whey. The curds are gathered together, without the whey, and put into cheese molds to help hold their shape. The molds are pressed tightly together to squeeze out any remaining whey. After the molds are removed, the cheese can be aged. Different kinds of cheese are made by varying the temperature during the process, as well as aging time, and including different types of bacteria and other additives that impart flavor to the cheese[2].

Curds and Whey
The whey that remains after the cheese is made is a thin, milky liquid. Whey is a very healthy food, containing all of the essential amino acids in an easily digestible form. It's an ingredient in many energy bars and supplements, and especially useful for athletes and others who would like to add extra protein to their diets. Of course, curds and whey is what Little Miss Muffet was eating in the famous nursery rhyme, too![2].

Here's a helpful video that shows how cheese is made. You can try this link: http://youtu.be/FP4aXT7iNxU or search YouTube for the title "Classic Sesame Street: How Cheese Is Made". (Even though it is from Sesame Street, older kids can benefit from watching it too.)

ACTIVITY: Mozzarella cheese is one of these simplest to make, and can easily be made in a home kitchen. You can search the internet or try this link for a recipe:
http://homecooking.about.com/od/cheeserecipes/r/bldairy22.htm

Yogurt
Did you know that you can heat milk to about 100 degrees for several hours to make your own yogurt? It's true! Yogurt is just milk where the naturally-occurring bacteria have been allowed to ferment. This changes the taste of the milk to the tangy flavor we associate with yogurt, and gives it a thicker texture. Fruit or sugar are often added to yogurt as well, but plain yogurt is simply milk that has been allowed to ferment[3]. If you'd like to try making your own yogurt, you can find a recipe here:
http://homecooking.about.com/od/dairyrecipes/r/bldairy7.htm or search for your own.

Finally, what does any of this have to do with nutrition? **Knowledge is power!** Know what you're eating, and how it was prepared. The best way to ensure you're eating healthy food is to make it yourself! Making homemade butter, cheese, or yogurt from natural ingredients is a wonderful way to stay healthy.

TRUE OR FALSE:

1. T / F   Buttermilk got its name because it is milk that contains a lot of butter.

2. T / F   Yogurt is made by adding the enzyme rennet to milk.

3. T / F   "Cultured buttermilk" is commercially produced buttermilk that contains added bacteria.

4. T / F   Whey is added to molds during the cheese making process.

5. T / F   Dairy products contain calcium, which your body needs for strong bones.

CRITICAL THINKING:

Imagine that you live on a farm, far away from any grocery stores, and you would like to surprise your mother by baking her a birthday cake. You look at the recipe and see that while you have most of the ingredients, you're missing the milk, eggs, and butter you need. You glance out at the barn and formulate a plan. What will you do in order to make the cake? Be sure to explain your plan step-by-step.

Optional - Additional Resources:

Here's a terrific video of kids making homemade yogurt:
http://watch.opb.org/video/1385917643/

Take this online calcium quiz to see if you're getting enough calcium each day:
http://www.dairycouncilofca.org/Tools/CalciumQuiz/

LESSON 15: EGGS

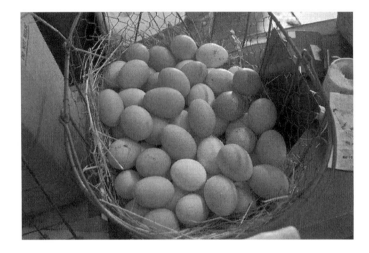

Not all eggs are created equal. In fact, they don't even all look the same. Of course, we've all seen the standard white eggs in the styrofoam cartons at the grocery store. But have you ever seen a brown egg? How about a blue one? **Ask any farmer - eggs come in all colors, depending on what breed of chicken they come from.** There are about 60 different breeds of chickens commonly found in the United States.

Egg-laying 101

Female chickens are called hens, and male chickens are called roosters. Hens lay eggs even if there are no roosters around to fertilize them. In fact, most **commercially sold eggs are unfertilized because chickens in large factory farms are never exposed to roosters at all.** The hens will lay an egg every day or so, depending on the characteristics of their breed, and if other conditions are right[1].

If roosters are present, as in some small farms or backyard chicken coops, there's a possibility that the eggs being laid have been fertilized. They can be held up to a bright light, in a process called "**candling**", to see if there's a developing embryo inside. Large chicken farms also use this process to check the eggs for dirt, cracks, and other imperfections before shipping them off to market. Even if you have both hens and roosters in your chicken coop, and the eggs may have been fertilized, **refrigerating the eggs just after they've been laid stops the development of any possible embryo** before its presence is even noticeable[1].

Chickens lay more eggs in the warmer months of the year, but not because of the temperature. They need about 14 hours of sunlight a day in order to lay eggs. The more sunlight, the more egg production increases. **There are fewer hours of sunlight in the winter, so many chickens will lay fewer eggs, or stop laying altogether if additional lighting is not provided**[1].

Pastured chickens vs. grain-fed chickens

Chickens raised on commercial egg farms often live in very cramped conditions, and may never even see real sunlight. The temperature is controlled, and artificial light is provided to get them to lay. These chickens rarely have access to the outdoors, and are usually fed grain rather than a normal chicken diet of grass and bugs. Their eggs are nowhere near as healthy as eggs from chickens who roam freely outside, eating fresh, green grass and catching bugs and worms for their meals[2,3]. As omnivores, that's what nature intended for chickens to eat!

You may notice that cartons of eggs in the store are sometimes labelled as being free-range, or cage-free. Some egg producers exploit loopholes in the law that allow them to label their eggs this way even if the bird has never been outdoors. If there is a small door in the chicken house somewhere that the bird could theoretically go through to access the outside, the producer can label their eggs in this way[4,5].

Not only are true free-range or pastured birds happier, but their eggs are of higher quality as well. These healthier eggs have higher levels of carotenoids, which are compounds the chickens get from eating fresh vegetation. The carotenoids make the egg yolk a thick, rich orange color, rather than the thin, yellow yolks from chickens who only eat grain[6].

Nutrients in eggs

If you compare the two types of eggs, the difference in the yolks is striking! Some egg producers have admitted to adding artificial coloring their eggs, to make the yolks look more orange in color, to entice people to continue buying them[7]. Seems dishonest, doesn't it?

The extra grass that a true free-range chicken eats translates into more nutrition in their eggs[8]. These eggs are much higher in Omega-3 fatty acids, which has huge health implications. The typical western diet is notoriously low in Omega-3 fats, and many people take a daily fish oil supplement in order to supplement their Omega-3 levels. Omega-3 fats are excellent for lowering cholesterol levels and risk for heart disease, diabetes, obesity, and depression[9].

Eggs from chickens confined indoors and fed grain have 20 times *less* Omega-3 than pastured chickens[8]. Have you seen labels on egg cartons claiming the eggs have increased levels of Omega-3? That's because those chickens' standard diet of grain was supplemented with fish meal (ground up fish) or they were fed flax seeds or soy[10]. And you thought you were just eating a simple egg!

Happier, healthier chickens produce more nutritious eggs. Besides Omega-3, pastured eggs also contain larger amounts of beta-carotene, lutein, vitamins A and E, and folic acid. And they taste better too!

ACTIVITY:
Buy some farm fresh pastured eggs and compare them to eggs from the supermarket. You can buy local eggs from a farmers market. Sometimes people will advertise eggs for sale in the Farm & Garden section of Craigslist. If you ask around in your circle of friends and family, you may even know someone who has chickens! Once you have some fresh, pastured eggs, you can compare one to an egg from the

grocery store. Make some notes and list their similarities and differences. Then crack the eggs into two separate bowls and compare them again. What do the yolks look like? Now cook the eggs and taste them. Which tastes better?

True or False:

1. T / F   Pastured chickens have lower levels of Omega-3 fatty acids than grain-fed chickens.

2. T / F   Most chickens on commercial egg farms are given a diet primarily of grain.

3. T / F   To tell if an egg is fertilized or not, you must first refrigerate it.

4. T / F   A hen will continue laying eggs every day or so, even without a rooster to fertilize them.

5. T / F   Chickens are herbivores.

Short answer questions:

1. If you crack an egg and find the yolk to be thin, runny, and pale yellow in color, what did the chicken who laid the egg likely eat?

2. Why do chickens lay fewer eggs in the winter months?

3. What is candling?

CRITICAL THINKING:

Skim over this research article published in the International Journal of Poultry Science. It describes an experiment to determine ways of coloring egg yolks to look darker orange, as if the chickens had been fed a more healthy diet of grasses[9].

http://www.pjbs.org/ijps/fin323.pdf   (Hint: Just read the "introduction" section of the article.)

1. What two agents are used to change the color of egg yolks?

2. Why do egg producers want to do this?

3. What is a natural way to achieve the desired color of egg yolk?

ADDITIONAL RESOURCES:

Here's a fun video about a chicken who has become a local celebrity in a small town in Mexico, because she lays green eggs! http://video.answers.com/chicken-lays-green-eggs-516911898 Why do you think this chicken lays green eggs?

Information and photos of different breeds of chickens
http://www.chickencrossing.org/breedlist.php

Learn what it takes to raise chickens yourself!
http://www.backyardchickens.com/

More on the nutrient content of eggs
http://nutritiondata.self.com/facts/dairy-and-egg-products/111/2

NUTRITION FOR HEALTHY KIDS

ANSWERS TO LESSONS 1-15

LESSON 1: ORGANIC TASTE TEST

ANSWERS:

1. True

2. False

3. True

4. False

5. True

Additional Activity:
Organic foods almost always cost more. Their production is more labor-intensive and sometimes it isn't possible to grow as many crops per acre as conventional produce.

LESSON 2: PLU CODES

ANSWERS

1. 3133
2. 94011
3. Sharlin
4. Red
5. 4048
6. it is genetically modified
7. bananas, peaches
8. 83087
9. 94400
10. 4523

1. The grapes would have a PLU code because they are sold by the pound and need to be weighed.

2. The PLU system is voluntary, and suppliers are not required to label genetically modified products. Some do label their GMOs, but many do not. The answer is "cannot be determined" because the corn could be an unlabeled GMO. (unless, of course, you live in an area that has made labelling of GMOs mandatory. Most of the United States does not require labelling.)

LESSON 3: GENETICALLY MODIFIED FOODS

TRUE/FALSE:
1. true
2. true

3. false
4. false
5. false

SHORT ANSWER:
1. Acceptable answers include soy, corn, canola, cotton, sugar beets. Other crops that are also found in GMO form, but less frequently, include papaya, yellow crookneck squash, and zucchini.

2. Acceptable answers include the following.
   1. allergies, sensitivity to other foods, immune reactions
   2. liver atrophy, toxicity, dysfunction
   3. infertility and reproductive abnormalities, lower birth weights, higher infant mortality
   4. general rates of disease and poor health

ACTIVITY:
This is not an exhaustive list of GMO products, but here are some examples of what you may find in your kitchen.
   Anything containing high fructose corn syrup (breads, prepackaged foods, soda)
   non-organic dairy products, unless labelled "non-rBST" or you know the manufacturer
      does not use rBST milk
   non-organic produce
   products containing corn or soy

Check the following list to help you find all the GMOs..

List of genetically modified foods:
It's virtually impossible to provide a complete list of genetically modified food (GM food) in the United States because there aren't any laws for genetically modified crops!
Some estimates say as many as 30,000 different products on grocery store shelves are *"modified."* That's largely because many processed foods contain soy. Half of North America's soy crop is genetically engineered!
Rapeseed - Resistance to certain pesticides and improved rapeseed cultivars to be free of erucic acid and glucosinolates. Gluconsinolates, which were found in rapeseed meal leftover from pressing, are toxic and had prevented the use of the meal in animal feed. In Canada, where "double-zero" rapeseed was developed, the crop was renamed "canola" (Canadian oil) to differentiate it from non-edible rapeseed.
Honey - can be produced from GM crops. Some Canadian honey comes from bees collecting nectar from GM canola plants. This has shut down exports of Canadian honey to Europe.
Cotton - Resistant to certain pesticides - considered a food because the oil can be consumed. The introduction of genetically engineered cotton plants has had an unexpectedly effect on Chinese agriculture. The so-called Bt cotton plants that produce a chemical that kills the cotton bollworm have not only reduced the incidence of the pest in cotton fields, but also in neighboring fields of corn, soybeans, and other crops.
Rice - Genetically modified to contain high amounts of Vitamin A. Rice containing human genes is to be grown in the US. Rather than end up on dinner plates, the rice will make human proteins useful for treating infant diarrhoea in the developing world.
Soybean - Genetically modified to be resistant to herbicides - Soy foods including, soy beverages, tofu, soy oil, soy flour, lecithin. Other products may include breads, pastries, snack foods, baked products, fried products, edible oil products and special purpose foods.

Sugar cane - Made resistant to certain pesticides. A large percentage of sweeteners used in processed food actually comes from corn, not sugar cane or beets. Genetically modified sugar cane is regarded so badly by consumers at the present time that it could not be marketed successfully.

Tomatoes - Made for a longer shelf life and to prevent a substance that causes tomatoes to rot and degrade.

Corn - Resistant to certain pesticides - Corn oil, flour, sugar or syrup. May include snack foods, baked goods, fried foods, edible oil products, confectionery, special purpose foods, and soft drinks.

Sweet corn - genetically modified to produces its own insecticide. Officials from the US Food and Drug Administration (FDA) have said that thousands of tonnes of genetically engineered sweetcorn have made their way into the human food supply chain, even though the produce has been approved only for use in animal feed. Recently Monsanto, a biotechnology food producer, said that about half of the USA's sweetcorn acreage has been planted with genetically modified seed this year.

Canola - Canola oil. May include edible oil products, fried foods, and baked products, snack foods.

Potatoes - (Atlantic, Russett Burbank, Russet Norkatah, and Shepody) - May include snack foods, processed potato products and other processed foods containing potatoes.

Flax - More and more food products contain flax oil and seed because of their excellent nutritional properties. No genetically modified flax is currently grown. An herbicide-resistant GM flax was introduced in 2001, but was soon taken off the market because European importers refused to buy it.

Papaya - The first virus resistant papayas were commercially grown in Hawaii in 1999. Transgenic papayas now cover about one thousand hectares, or three quarters of the total Hawaiian papaya crop. Monsanto, donated technology to Tamil Nadu Agricultural University, Coimbatore, for developing a papaya resistant to the ringspot virus in India.

Squash - (yellow crookneck) - Some zucchini and yellow crookneck squash are also GM but they are not popular with farmers.

Red-hearted chicory - (radicchio) - Chicory (Cichorium intybus var. foliosum) is popular in some regions as a salad green, especially in France and Belgium. Scientists developed a genetically modified line of chicory containing a gene that makes it male sterile, simply facilitating the production of hybrid cultivars. Today there is no genetically modified chicory on the market.

Cotton seed oil - Cottonseed oil and linters. Products may include blended vegetable oils, fried foods, baked foods, snack foods, edible oil products, and smallgoods casings.

Tobacco -The company Vector has a GMO tobacco being sold under the brand of Quest® cigarettes in the U.S. It is engineered to produce low or no nicotine.

Meat - Meat and dairy products usually come from animals that have eaten GM feed.

Peas - Genetically modified (GM) peas created immune responses in mice, suggesting that they may also create serious allergic reactions in people. The peas had been inserted with a gene from kidney beans, which creates a protein that acts as a pesticide.

Vegetable Oil - Most generic vegetable oils and margarines used in restaurants and in processed foods in North America are made from soy, corn, canola, or cottonseed. Unless these oils specifically say "Non-GMO" or "Organic," it is probably genetically modified.

Sugarbeets - May include any processed foods containing sugar.

Dairy Products - About 22 percent of cows in the U.S. are injected with recombinant (genetically modified) bovine growth hormone (rbGH).

Vitamins - Vitamin C (ascorbic acid) is often made from corn, vitamin E is usually made from soy. Vitamins A, B2, B6, and B12 may be derived from GMOs as well as vitamin D and vitamin K may have "carriers" derived from GM corn sources, such as starch, glucose, and maltodextrin.

This list is from: http://www.disabled-world.com/fitness/gm-foods.php#ixzz1LcYkb5fO

CRITICAL THINKING QUESTION:
Studies have not yet been done on this matter, so this is purely a hypothetical question to get kids thinking about the possibilities, and the realize the dangers of ingesting something that hasn't been thoroughly tested. The answer is that your intestinal cells would start producing their own supply of pesticide, which would likely poison your body!

LESSON 4: USDA ORGANIC

TRUE or FALSE:

1. False

2. True

3. False

4. False

5. True

LABEL READING EXERCISE:
The salsa, ranch dressing, and oats are all USDA organic. The beef broth does not have the USDA organic seal on its label.

LESSON 5: SWEETENERS - SUCRALOSE

Simply compare the two chemicals structures shown at the beginning of this assignment and determine where the 3 -OH (or -HO) groups have been replaced by Cl in the second drawing.

TRUE OR FALSE:

1. False
2. False
3. False
4. True
5. False

LESSON 6: SWEETENERS - ASPARTAME

TRUE OR FALSE:

1. True
2. True
3. False
4. False

5. True

SHORT ANSWER QUESTIONS:

If autopsy were delayed, decomposition would make identifying a cause of death nearly impossible.

Removal of tumors would artificially lower the cancer risk being reported.

ACTIVITY:

Although the weight of sugar (or more commonly, high fructose corn syrup) and aspartame are not that different, aspartame is much sweeter than sugar/HFCS. Less aspartame is needed to sweeten the diet soda than sugar/HFCS needed to sweeten the regular soda. The can of diet soda weighs less, and will float.

LESSON 7: HIGH FRUCTOSE CORN SYRUP

TRUE OR FALSE:

1. True
2. False
3. True
4. False
5. False

GRAPH QUESTIONS:

1. approx. 23-24%
2. approx. 20% more
3. B
4. 30 lbs.
5. HFCS consumption started to fall.

LESSON 8: PRODUCE - FROM SEED TO TABLE

1. Yes. The longer the distance your food has traveled, the less likely it is to be fresh.

2. No. The food miles will only tell you how much energy was used to transport the food, not how much energy was used to grow it.

3. reduce greenhouse gas emissions from the transport of food long distances, support the local economy, to foster a sense of community among neighbors, fresher food

4. No.

5. trucks, trains, ships

6. Each type of fruit or vegetable grows best in a certain climate, and with particular soil conditions, rainfall amounts, etc.

7. Strawberries are picked by hand to avoid crushing them with large equipment.

8. Corn

9. Corn

10. October

Most soybeans are grown in the upper mid-west. They do not grow well in the south, or west, or in areas of the country that are too hot and dry.

LESSON 9: BASIC BOTANY OF EDIBLE PLANTS

1. photosynthesis

2. The roots absorb water from the soil.

3. Autotrophic means something can produce its own food, like plants can!

4. dandelions

5. If you aren't sure about the safety of a plant, do not touch or eat it. Ask a parent. It's best to not eat wild plants at all without your parent's permission.

ACTIVITY:
Here are some to get you started!

    Fruits - tomatoes, peppers, pears, apples, squash
    Roots - carrots, yams, radishes, potatoes, sweet potatoes, beets
    Seeds - peas, nuts, berries, corn, sunflower seeds
    Leaves - lettuce, cabbage, spinach
    Stems - asparagus, celery
    Flowers - broccoli, cauliflower

LESSON 10: SUSTAINABLE FARMING

SHORT ANSWER:

1. Green manure refers to crops like alfalfa and several types of legumes (beans) that are grown only to be plowed under and provide nutrients like nitrogen to replenish the soil.

2. Preserving the habitat of bees, wild birds, and butterflies will help attract them to the land. Many of these are beneficial as pollinators, and useful to attract other forms of wildlife to the farm too.

3. nitrogen, phosphorus, potassium, magnesium, calcium

4. Being a good steward of the land means to preserve the ecology and natural habitats present, and to use the land wisely so it will continue to produce well.

5. An insecticide kills unwanted insects.

TRUE OR FALSE:

1. false

2. false

3. true

4. false

5. false

LESSON 11: GRASS-FED AND PASTURED MEATS

TRUE OR FALSE:

1. true
2. false
3. false
4. false
5. true

SHORT ANSWER:
1. Cows eat mainly grass. Chickens eat plants and bugs.
2. Fat is high in calories, and grass-fed meats are lower in fat, so they're lower in calories too.

MULTIPLE CHOICE:
1. E
2. A
3. E
4. E
5. C

LESSON 12: LIFE CYCLES AND ANIMAL HUSBANDRY BASICS

TRUE OR FALSE:

1. True
2. True
3. True

4. True
5. False

CRITICAL THINKING EXERCISES:

1. There are several acceptable options. You could arrange for a male from another zoo to be brought to your zoo to mate with the female, or you could arrange for someone to catch a male leopard in the wild for the same purpose. Artificial insemination is the most likely option, by collecting sperm from a male leopard at another zoo and sending it to your zoo.

2. Both of these options would work, but the most cost-efficient choice would be artificially inseminating your female cows with the sperm of the bull at the neighboring farm.

3. 1) 60 pigs
   2) 200/mo + 40 = 240/mo
   3) $1,000
   4) It costs $240/mo to raise 60 pigs, so each pig costs $4/mo. To raise one pig for 6 months would be 6 x 4 = 24.
   5) $100 sales price - $24 = $76 profit

<u>Suggestion for the younger kids:</u> To keep the little ones busy, try teaching them songs like "The Farmer in the Dell" or "Old MacDonald". You could also make a matching game where the kids match adult animals with their babies, such as pigs and piglets, cows and calves, or a sheep and lamb.

LESSON 13: DAIRY - WHAT IS PASTEURIZATION?

TRUE OR FALSE:

1. False
2. False
3. True
4. False
5. True

SHORT ANSWER:

1. pasteurization = 161.5 degrees for 15 seconds
   UHT pasteurization = 285 degrees for 1-2 seconds

2. Our bodies are home to numerous kinds of beneficial bacteria that help us digest food, keep the harmful bacteria in check, and even aid our immune systems to keep us healthy.

CRITICAL THINKING:

A hand crank was used to spin the container. The centrifugal force created would send the heavier milk to the walls of the container, and the lighter cream would end up in the center. Each would travel down a spout into separate containers.

LESSON 14: DAIRY - CHEESE, BUTTER, MILK, CURDS & WHEY, BUTTERMILK, YOGURT

TRUE OR FALSE:

1. False
2. False
3. True
4. False
5. True

CRITICAL THINKING:

You can get eggs from chickens in the barn, and you can get milk from the dairy cow. You'll need to skim the cream from the milk and make butter out of it. If you don't have an electric mixer, you could use an old-fashioned butter churn to make the butter. Be sure to save the buttermilk for later!

LESSON 15: EGGS

TRUE OR FALSE:

1. false
2. true
3. false
4. true
5. false

SHORT ANSWER:

1. grain
2. Chickens need about 14 hours per day of sunlight to lay eggs, and there is less sunlight in the winter.
3. Candling is the process of holding an egg up to a bright light to determine if there is a chick inside, or to check for cracks and other imperfections.

CRITICAL THINKING:

1. marigolds (a type of yellow or orange flower) and orange peels
2. Egg producers know that many consumers prefer an orange colored egg yolk because it means the chicken ate plenty of healthy grasses and bugs, and the egg will be healthier too. Producers try to fool consumers by altering the color of the yolk, while keeping the chicken on a cheaper diet of grain.
3. Pastured chickens who eat grass, weeds, insects, and worms, the natural diet of a chicken, will have darker, orange egg yolks naturally.

© 2014 Jennifer Needham / Nutrition For Healthy Kids

References

Lesson 1: Organic Taste Test

1. Van Loo EJ, Caputo V, Nayga RM, Meullenet JF, Ricke SC. Consumers' willingness to pay for organic chicken breast: Evidence from choice experiment. Food Quality and Preference. 2011 Oct;22(7):603-13.
2. Chhabra R, Kolli S, Bauer JH. Organically grown food provides health benefits to Drosophila melanogaster. PLoS One. 2013;8(1):e52988.
3. USDA releases organic food guidelines. J Am Vet Med Assoc. 2001 Feb 15;218(4):489.
4. Kramkowska M, Grzelak T, Czyżewska K. Benefits and risks associated with genetically modified food products. Ann Agric Environ Med. 2013;20(3):413-9.
5. Vecchio L, Cisterna B, Malatesta M, Martin TE, Biggiogera M. Eur J Histochem. Ultrastructural analysis of testes from mice fed on genetically modified soybean. 2004 Oct-Dec;48(4):448-54.
6. A. Pusztai and S. Bardocz, "GMO in animal nutrition: potential benefits and risks," Chapter 17, Biology of Nutrition in Growing Animals, R. Mosenthin, J. Zentek and T. Zebrowska (Eds.) Elsevier, October 2005
7. Yum HY, Lee SY, Lee KE, Sohn MH, Kim KE. Genetically modified and wild soybeans: an immunologic comparison. Allergy Asthma Proc. 2005 May-Jun;26(3):210-6.
8. Irina Ermakova, "Genetically modified soy leads to the decrease of weight and high mortality of rat pups of the first generation. Preliminary studies," Ecosinform 1 (2006): 4–9.
9. Petrariu FD, Gavăt V, Cozma AG. Current issues regarding organic food. Rev Med Chir Soc Med Nat Iasi. 2005 Oct-Dec;109(4):866-70.
10. Palupi E, Jayanegara A, Ploeger A, Kahl J. Comparison of nutritional quality between conventional and organic dairy products: a meta-analysis. J Sci Food Agric. 2012 Nov;92(14):2774-81.
11. Toschi TG, Bendini A, Barbieri S, Valli E, Cezanne ML, Buchecker K, Canavari M. Organic and conventional nonflavored yogurts from the Italian market: study on sensory profiles and consumer acceptability. J Sci Food Agric. 2012 Nov;92(14):2788-95.

Lesson 2: PLU Codes

1. International Federation for Produce Standards homepage [internet]. International Federation for Produce Standards. [cited 2014 Mar]. Available from: http://www.ifpsglobal.com
2. Poll: Skepticism of Genetically Modified Foods [internet]. ABC News. [updated 2013 Jun 19; cited 2014 Apr 20]. Available from: http://abcnews.go.com/Technology/story?id=97567
3. User's Guide: Produce PLU Codes [internet]. International Federation for Produce Standards. [updated 2012; cited 2014 Mar]. Available from: http://www.plucodes.com/docs/Users_Guide.pdf

Lesson 3: Genetically Modified Foods

1. Celec P, Kukucková M, Renczésová V, Natarajan S, Pálffy R, Gardlík R, Hodosy J, Behuliak M, Vlková B, Minárik G, Szemes T, Stuchlík S, Turna J. Biological and biomedical aspects of genetically modified food. Biomed Pharmacother. 2005 Dec;59(10):531-40.
2. Diels J, Cunha M, Manaia C, Sabugosa-Madeira B, Silva M. Association of financial or professional conflict of interest to research outcomes on health risks or nutritional assessment studies of genetically modified products. Food Policy. 2011 April;36(2)197–203.

3. de Vendômois JS, Cellier D, Vélot C, Clair E, Mesnage R, Séralini GE.Int J Biol Sci. Debate on GMOs health risks after statistical findings in regulatory tests. 2010 Oct 5;6(6):590-8.
4. US Food and Drug Administration. Statement of policy: Foods derived from new plant varieties. FDA Federal Register. 29 May 1992; 57(104): 229.
5. Kramkowska M, Grzelak T, Czyżewska K. Benefits and risks associated with genetically modified food products. Ann Agric Environ Med. 2013;20(3):413-9.
6. Bawa AS, Anilakumar KR. Genetically modified foods: safety, risks and public concerns-a review. J Food Sci Technol. 2013 Dec;50(6):1035-1046.
7. van den Eede G, Aarts H, Buhk HJ, Corthier G, Flint HJ, Hammes W, Jacobsen B, Midtvedt T, van der Vossen J, von Wright A, Wackernagel W, Wilcks A. The relevance of gene transfer to the safety of food and feed derived from genetically modified (GM) plants. Food Chem Toxicol. 2004 Jul;42(7):1127-56.
8. 20 Questions About Genetically Modified Foods [internet]. World Health Organization. [updated 2014; cited 2014 Apr 3]. Available from: http://www.who.int/foodsafety/publications/biotech/20questions/en/
9. Stelwagen K, Verrinfer-Gibbins AM, McBride BW. Applications of recombinant DNA technology to improve milk production: a review. Livestock Production Science. 1992 June;31(3-4):153-178.
10. Molento CM, Block E, Cue RI, Lacasse P, Petitclerc D. Effects of insulin, recombinant bovine somatotropin (rbST) and their interaction on DMI and milk fat production in dairy cows. Livestock Production Science. 2005 Nov;97(2-3);173-182.
11. Jurkiewicz A, Zagórski J, Bujak F, Lachowski S, Florek-Łuszczki M. Emotional attitudes of young people completing secondary schools towards genetic modification of organisms (GMO) and genetically modified foods (GMF). Ann Agric Environ Med. 2014 Mar 31;21(1):205-11.
12. Netherwood T, Martín-Orúe SM, O'Donnell AG, Gockling S, Graham J, Mathers JC, Gilbert HJ. Assessing the survival of transgenic plant DNA in the human gastrointestinal tract. Nat Biotechnol. 2004 Feb;22(2):204-9.

Lesson 4: USDA Organic

1. USDA releases organic food guidelines. J Am Vet Med Assoc. 2001 Feb 15;218(4):489.
2. USDA Organic Program [internet]. United States Department of Agriculture, Agricultural Marketing Service. [updated 2014 Jan 15; cited 2014 Apr 22]. Available from: http://www.ams.usda.gov/AMSv1.0/nop
3. USDA Organic Program: Organic Certification and Accreditation [internet]. United States Department of Agriculture, Agricultural Marketing Service. [updated 2012 Dec 31; cited 2014 Apr 22]. Available from: http://www.ams.usda.gov/AMSv1.0/ams.fetchTemplateData.do?template=TemplateN&navID=NationalOrganicProgram&leftNav=NationalOrganicProgram&page=NOPAccreditationandCertification&description=Accreditation%20and%20Certification&acct=nopgeninfo

Lesson 5: Sweeteners – Sucralose

1. Burkhard Bilger, Department of Food Science, "The Search for Sweet," The New Yorker, May 22, 2006, p. 40.
2. Knight I. The development and applications of sucralose, a new high-intensity sweetener. Can J Physiol Pharmacol. 1994 Apr;72(4):435-9.

3. Schiffman SS, Rother KI. Sucralose, a synthetic organochlorine sweetener: overview of biological issues. J Toxicol Environ Health B Crit Rev. 2013;16(7):399-451.
4. Roberts A, Renwick AG, Sims J, Snodin DJ. Sucralose metabolism and pharmacokinetics in man. Food Chem Toxicol. 2000;38 Suppl 2:S31-41.
5. Sims J, Roberts A, Daniel JW, Renwick AG. Food Chem Toxicol. The metabolic fate of sucralose in rats. 2000;38 Suppl 2:S115-21.
6. Abou-Donia MB, El-Masry EM, Abdel-Rahman AA, McLendon RE, Schiffman SS. Splenda alters gut microflora and increases intestinal p-glycoprotein and cytochrome p-450 in male rats. J Toxicol Environ Health A. 2008;71(21):1415-29.
7. Turner, James. FDA amends regulations that include sucralose as a non-nutritive sweetener in food [internet]. FDA Consumer. 2006 Apr 3. Retrieved 2014 Apr 8. Available from: http://www.fda.gov/ohrms/dockets/dockets/06p0158/06p-0158-cp00001-01-vol1.pdf.
8. de Araujo IE, Lin T, Veldhuizen MG, Small DM. Metabolic regulation of brain response to food cues. Curr Biol. 2013 May 20;23(10):878-83.
9. Swithers SE. Artificial sweeteners produce the counterintuitive effect of inducing metabolic derangements. Trends Endocrinol Metab. 2013 Sep;24(9):431-41.
10. CFR – Code of Federal Regulations Title 21 [internet]. U.S. Food and Drug Administration. 2011-04-01. Retrieved 18 March 2014. Available from: http://www.accessdata.fda.gov/scripts/cdrh/cfdocs/cfcfr/CFRSearch.cfm?fr=101.60.
11. AlDeeb OA, Mahgoub H, Foda NH. Sucralose. Profiles Drug Subst Excip Relat Methodol. 2013;38:423-62.

Lesson 6: Sweeteners – Aspartame

1. Roberts, HJ. Aspartame Disease: An Ignored Epidemic. Sunshine Sentinel Press; 2001.
2. Soffritti M, Padovani M, Tibaldi E, Falcioni L, Manservisi F, Belpoggi F. The carcinogenic effects of aspartame: The urgent need for regulatory re-evaluation. Am J Ind Med. 2014 Apr;57(4):383-97.
3. Whitehouse CR, Boullata J, McCauley LA. The potential toxicity of artificial sweeteners. AAOHN J. 2008 Jun;56(6):251-9; quiz 260-1.
4. Smith RJ. Aspartame approved despite risks. Science. 1981 Aug 28;213(4511):986-7.
5. Cooper JR, Kini MM. Biochemical aspects of methanol poisoning. Biochem Pharmacol. 1962 Jun;11:405-16.
6. Maher TJ, Wurtman RJ. Possible neurologic effects of aspartame, a widely used food additive. Environ Health Perspect. 1987 Nov;75:53-7.
7. Janssen PJ, van der Heijden CA. Aspartame: review of recent experimental and observational data. Toxicology. 1988 Jun;50(1):1-26.
8. Potenza DP, el-Mallakh RS. Aspartame: clinical update. Conn Med. 1989 Jul;53(7):395-400.
9. Sturtevant FM. Use of aspartame in pregnancy. Int J Fertil. 1985;30(1):85-7.
10. Horio Y, Sun Y, Liu C, Saito T, Kurasaki M. Environ Toxicol Pharmacol. Aspartame-induced apoptosis in PC12 cells. 2014 Jan;37(1):158-65.
11. Huff J, LaDou J. Aspartame bioassay findings portend human cancer hazards. Int J Occup Environ Health. 2007 Oct-Dec;13(4):446-8.
12. The Bressler Report: Actual Text of an FDA Report on Searle. Cited 2014 Mar 30. Available from: http://dorway.com/history-of-aspartame/the-bressler-report/.

Lesson 7: Sweeteners – High Fructose Corn Syrup

1. Kramkowska M, Grzelak T, Czyżewska K. Benefits and risks associated with genetically modified food products. Ann Agric Environ Med. 2013;20(3):413-9.

2. Dufault R, Schnoll R, Lukiw WJ, Leblanc B, Cornett C, Patrick L, Wallinga D, Gilbert SG, Crider R. Mercury exposure, nutritional deficiencies and metabolic disruptions may affect learning in children. Behav Brain Funct. 2009 Oct 27;5:44.
3. Dufault R, LeBlanc B, Schnoll R, Cornett C, Schweitzer L, Wallinga D, Hightower J, Patrick L, Lukiw WJ. Mercury from chlor-alkali plants: measured concentrations in food product sugar. Environ Health. 2009 Jan 26;8:2.
4. Study Finds High-Fructose Corn Syrup Contains Mercury. Washington Post [internet] 2009 Jan 28; cited 2014 Feb 10. Available from: http://www.washingtonpost.com/wp-dyn/content/article/2009/01/26/AR2009012601831.html.
5. Akram M, Hamid A. Mini review on fructose metabolism. Obes Res Clin Pract. 2013 Mar-Apr;7(2):e89-e94.
6. Riveros MJ, Parada A, Pettinelli P. Fructose consumption and its health implications; fructose malabsorption and nonalcoholic fatty liver disease. Nutr Hosp. 2014 Mar 1;29(3):491-9.
7. Kelishadi R, Mansourian M, Heidari-Beni M. Association of fructose consumption and components of metabolic syndrome in human studies: A systematic review and meta-analysis. Nutrition. 2014 May;30(5):503-510.
8. Shapiro A, Mu W, Roncal C, Cheng KY, Johnson RJ, Scarpace PJ. Fructose-induced leptin resistance exacerbates weight gain in response to subsequent high-fat feeding. Am J Physiol Regul Integr Comp Physiol. 2008 Nov;295(5):R1370-5.
9. White JS. Straight talk about high-fructose corn syrup: what it is and what it ain't. Am J Clin Nutr. 2008 Dec;88(6):1716S-1721S.
10. Bray GA, Nielsen SJ, Popkin BM. Consumption of high-fructose corn syrup in beverages may play a role in the epidemic of obesity. Am J Clin Nutr. 2004 Apr;79(4):537-43.
11. Liu H, Huang D, McArthur DL, Boros LG, Nissen N, Heaney AP. Fructose induces transketolase flux to promote pancreatic cancer growth. Cancer Res. 2010 Aug 1;70(15):6368-76.
12. Port AM, Ruth MR, Istfan NW. Fructose consumption and cancer: is there a connection? Curr Opin Endocrinol Diabetes Obes. 2012 Oct;19(5):367-74.
13. How Sweet It Isn't: Cutting Through The Hype and Deception. [internet]. Alliance For Natural Health. 2011 Feb 8; Cited 2014 Mar 3. Available from: http://www.anh-usa.org/how-sweet-it-isnt-cutting-through-the-hype-and-deception/.
14. Bray GA. Fructose: should we worry? Int J Obes (Lond). 2008 Dec;32 Suppl 7:S127-31
15. Land a, MM. Response to Petition from Corn Refiners Association to Authorize "Corn Sugar" as an Alternate Common or Usual Name for High Fructose Corn Syrup (HFCS) [internet]. US Food and Drug Administration. [updated 2012 May 12; cited 2014 Mar 28]. Available from: http://www.fda.gov/aboutFDA/CentersOffices/OfficeofFoods/CFSAN/CFSANFOIAElectronicReadingRoom/ucm305226.htm
16. Sobel LL, Dalby E. Sugar or high fructose corn syrup-what should nurses teach patients and families? Worldviews Evid Based Nurs. 2014 Apr;11(2):126-32.

Lesson 8: Produce – From Seed to Table

1. Young EM, Fors SW, Hayes DM. Associations between Perceived Parent Behaviors and Middle School Student Fruit and Vegetable Consumption. J Nutr Educ Behav. 2004 Jan-Feb;36(1):2-8.
2. Food Miles Calculator. [internet] Food Miles. Cited 2014 Apr 4. Available from: http://www.foodmiles.com/.
3. Major Crops Grown in the United States. [internet] US Environmental Protection Agency. Updated 2013 Apr 11; Cited 2014 Feb 26. Available from: http://www.epa.gov/oecaagct/ag101/cropmajor.html.

4. Food Miles. [internet] Farmscape Ecology Program at Hawthorne Valley Farm. Cited 2013 May 25. Available from: http://hawthornevalleyfarm.org/fep/foodmiles.html.

Lesson 9: Produce – Basic Botany of Edible Plants

1. Gibbs L, Staiger PK, Johnson B, Block K, Macfarlane S, Gold L, Kulas J, Townsend M, Long C, Ukoumunne O. Expanding children's food experiences: the impact of a school-based kitchen garden program. J Nutr Educ Behav. 2013 Mar;45(2):137-46.
2. Heim S, Stang J, Ireland M. A garden pilot project enhances fruit and vegetable consumption among children. J Am Diet Assoc. 2009 Jul;109(7):1220-6.
3. Edible Wild Food. [internet] Cited 2013 Nov 11. Available from: http://www.ediblewildfood.com.
4. Potato Plant Poisoning: Green Tubers and Sprouts. [internet] Medline Plus. Updated 2011 Dec 15. Cited 2013 Oct 12. Available from: http://www.nlm.nih.gov/medlineplus/ency/article/002875.htm.
5. Rhubarb Leaves Poisoning. [internet] Medline Plus. Updated 2011 Dec 15. Cited 2013 Oct 12. Available from: http://www.nlm.nih.gov/medlineplus/ency/article/002876.htm.
6. Reynolds T. Hemlock alkaloids from Socrates to poison aloes. Phytochemistry. 2005 Jun;66(12):1399–1406.

Lesson 10: Sustainable Farming

1. Hughes LJ. Creating a farm and food learning box curriculum for preschool-aged children and their families. J Nutr Educ Behav. 2007 May-Jun;39(3):171-2.
2. Aarestrup F. Sustainable farming: Get pigs off antibiotics. Nature 486, 465–466 (28 June 2012).
3. Filipiak J. The work of local culture: Wendell Berry and communities as the source of farming knowledge. Agric Hist. 2011;85(2):174-94.
4. Robinson-O'Brien R, Larson N, Neumark-Sztainer D, Hannan P. Characteristics and dietary patterns of adolescents who value eating locally grown, organic, nongenetically engineered, and nonprocessed food. J Nutr Educ Behav. 2009 Jan-Feb;41(1):11-8.
5. Companion Planting: The Three Sisters. [internet] The Old Farmer's Almanac. Cited 2014 Jan 24. Available from: http://www.almanac.com/content/companion-planting-three-sisters.

Lesson 11: Meat – Grass fed and Pastured Meats

1. Ponte PI, Alves SP, Bessa RJ, Ferreira LM, Gama LT, Brás JL, Fontes CM, Prates JA. Influence of pasture intake on the fatty acid composition, and cholesterol, tocopherols, and tocotrienols content in meat from free-range broilers. Poult Sci. 2008 Jan;87(1):80-8.
2. Bourre JM. Where to find omega-3 fatty acids and how feeding animals with diet enriched in omega-3 fatty acids to increase nutritional value of derived products for human: what is actually useful ? J Nutr Health Aging. 2005 Jul-Aug;9(4):232-42.
3. Swanson D, Block R, Mousa SA. Omega-3 fatty acids EPA and DHA: health benefits throughout life. Adv Nutr. 2012 Jan;3(1):1-7.
4. Daley CA, Abbott A, Doyle PS, Nader GA, Larson S. A review of fatty acid profiles and antioxidant content in grass-fed and grain-fed beef. Nutr J. 2010 Mar 10;9:10.
5. Tobias I, Ndubuisi E, Uchechi E, Chika O. Waste to Wealth- Value Recovery from Agrofood Processing Wastes Using Biotechnology: A Review. British Biotechnology Journal 4(4): 418-481, 2014.
6. Decoding Food Labels. [internet] Tufts University Office of Sustainability. Updated 2008. Cited 2014 Mar 27. Available from: http://sustainability.tufts.edu/decoding-food-labels/.

Lesson 12: Meat – Life Cycles and Animal Husbandry Basics

1. Lukefahr SD. Teaching international animal agriculture. J Anim Sci. 1999 Nov;77(11):3106-13.
2. Agricultural Education [internet]. Future Farmers of America. [updated 2014; cited 2014 Apr]. Available from: https://www.ffa.org/About/WhoWeAre/Pages/AgriculturalEducation.aspx.
3. Ellis C, Irvine L. Reproducing Dominion: Emotional Apprenticeship in the 4-H Youth Livestock Program. Society & Animals. 2010;18(1):21 – 39.

Lesson 13: Dairy – What is Pasteurization?

1. Macdonald LE, Brett J, Kelton D, Majowicz SE, Snedeker K, Sargeant JM. A systematic review and meta-analysis of the effects of pasteurization on milk vitamins, and evidence for raw milk consumption and other health-related outcomes. J Food Prot. 2011 Nov;74(11):1814-32.
2. Ijaz, N. Unpasteurized Milk: Myths and Evidence. Grand Rounds Presentation, BC Centers for Disease Control; 2013 May 16; Vancouver, BC, Canada.
3. Raw milk expert testimony dated: April 25, 2008 Case: ORGANIC PASTURES DAIRY COMPANY, LLC, and CLARAVALE FARM, INC., Plaintiffs, vs. No. CU-07-00204 STATE OF CALIFORNIA and A.G. KAWAMURA, SECRETARY OF CALIFORNIA DEPARTMENT OF FOOD AND AGRICULTURE, Defendants. - Expert Witnesses: Dr. Theodore Beals & Dr. Ronald Hull.
4. Pasteurization: Definition and Methods [internet]. International Dairy Foods Association. [updated 2009 Jun; cited 2014 Mar]. Available from: http://www.idfa.org/docs/default-source/resource-library/249_pasteurization-definition-and-methods.pdf?sfvrsn=2.
5. Eng, J. [Internet]. NBC News. [updated 2012 Feb 15; cited 2014 Mar 12]. Available from: http://usnews.nbcnews.com/_news/2012/02/15/10418406-amish-farmer-targeted-by-fda-raids-shuts-down-raw-milk-business?lite
6. Giacometti F, Bonilauri P, Serraino A, Peli A, Amatiste S, Arrigoni N, Bianchi M, Bilei S, Cascone G, Comin D, Daminelli P, Decastelli L, Fustini M, Mion R, Petruzzelli A, Rosmini R, Rugna G, Tamba M, Tonucci F, Bolzoni G. Four-year monitoring of foodborne pathogens in raw milk sold by vending machines in Italy. J Food Prot. 2013 Nov;76(11):1902-7.

Lesson 14: Dairy – Cheese, Butter, Milk, Curds & Whey, Buttermilk, and Yogurt

1. Schmutz PH, Vines DT, Hoyle EH. Safe Handling of Milk and Dairy Products [internet]. Clemson University Cooperative Extension Office. [updated 2007 Mar; cited 2014 Mar 29]. Available from: http://www.clemson.edu/extension/hgic/food/pdf/hgic3510.pdf
2. Flores, NC. Making Homemade Cheese [internet]. Cooperative Extension Service of the College of Agriculture and Home Economics, New Mexico State University. [updated 2013 Jun; cited 2014 Mar 30]. Available from: http://aces.nmsu.edu/pubs/_e/E-216.pdf
3. Cascio J, Dinstel RR. Making Yogurt at Home [internet]. University of Alaska Cooperative Extension Service. [updated 2013 Sep 27; cited 2014 Mar 19]. Available from: http://www.uaf.edu/files/ces/publications-db/catalog/hec/FNH-00062.pdf.

Lesson 15: Eggs

1. Clauer, PJ. Proper Handling of Eggs: From Hen to Consumption [internet]. Virginia Cooperative Extension of Virginia Polytechnic Institute and Virginia State University. [updated 2009; cited 2014 Mar 21]. Available from: http://pubs.ext.vt.edu/2902/2902-1091/2902-1091_pdf.pdf.
2. Guesdon V and Faure JM. Laying performance and egg quality in hens kept in standard or furnished cages. Animal Research 2004 53:45-57.
3. Rodenburg TB, Tuyttens FM, and Sonck B. Welfare, health, and hygiene of laying hens housed in furnished cages and in alternative housing systems. Journal of Applied Animal Welfare Science 2005 8(3):211-26.
4. How To Read Egg Carton Labels [internet]. Humane Society of the United States. [updated 2013 Apr 10; cited 2014 Mar 30]. Available from: http://www.humanesociety.org/issues/confinement_farm/facts/guide_egg_labels.html.
5. National Organic Program [internet]. Agricultural Marketing Service of the United States Department of Agriculture. [updated 2012 Oct 17; cited 2014 Mar 29]. Available from: http://www.ams.usda.gov/AMSv1.0/ams.fetchTemplateData.do?template=TemplateC&leftNav=NationalOrganicProgram&page=NOPConsumers&description=Consumers
6. Bourre JM. Effect of increasing the omega-3 fatty acid in the diets of animals on the animal products consumed by humans. Med Sci (Paris). 2005 Aug-Sep;21(8-9):773-9.
7. Hasin BM, Ferdaus AM, Islam MA, Uddin MJ, and Islam MS. Marigold and Orange Skin as Egg Yolk Color Promoting Agents. International Journal of Poultry Science 5 (10): 979-987, 2006.
8. Simopoulos AP. New products from the agri-food industry: the return of n-3 fatty acids into the food supply. Lipids 1999;34 Suppl:S297-301.
9. Swanson D, Block R, Mousa SA. Omega-3 fatty acids EPA and DHA: health benefits throughout life. Adv Nutr. 2012 Jan;3(1):1-7.
10. Bean LD, Leeson S. Long-term effects of feeding flaxseed on performance and egg fatty acid composition of brown and white hens. Poult Sci. 2003 Mar;82(3):388-94.

ABOUT THE AUTHOR

Jennifer Needham is a homeschooling mom to six incredible kids. Teaching others about nutrition is her passion, because people can't be expected to eat right if they aren't taught *how*!

Jennifer has a master's degree in Nutrition, a bachelor's degree in Biology, and a professional background in healthcare. She works from home writing science curriculum and doing freelance work in both education and nutrition. She also teaches nutrition classes for homeschoolers, both online and in her local area.

For additional nutrition lessons, articles for parents, and more teaching resources, visit her website at www.NutritionForHealthyKids.com

Made in the USA
Charleston, SC
29 September 2014